DENTAL *DELIRIUM*: A "HUMOROUS" LOOK AT DENTISTRY

Acknowledgments

*I wish to thank all those in my personal and
scholastic lives who made this book possible.*

Mr. Nick Productions, LLC
©2021 by Mr. Nick Productions, LLC

Edited by my longtime friend and editor/writer,
Marilyn Milow Francis – Thank you

Front cover art – Dr. Mayputz and Kristy Klein
Back cover and spine – Dr. Mayputz and Kristy Klein
Book layout – Kristy Klein | FifteenBlue.com

Photo of pickleball player – Anonymous
Published by Mr. Nick Productions, LLC ©2021

This book was NOT written by a ghostwriter

ISBN: 978-0-578-86267-5

Dedications

To all the dental assistants that have worked on patients with me over the years while putting up with my personality – thank you! And a very special shout out and sincere thank-you to the best of the best: there are dental assistants and then there is Tanya A.! Those seven years working together were the most professional, satisfying and fun-filled times of my dental career.

And to my lovely and multi-talented daughter Brigette, whose irreverent and eclectic sense of humor rivals my own. Although you would have made a brilliant dentist, you wisely chose not to follow in my footsteps. Instead, you followed your heart and passion. Your subsequent doctorate degree in entomology was well-earned and made me a proud papa. You know it!

Preface

There is already a myriad of annoying and cloying books allegedly depicting humorous dental situations. Those books are actually bereft of honest storytelling and feature spineless and whimsical dentists who do not want to "rock the boat" and only gently poke fun at the dental field. The highbrow comedy, tongue-in-cheek teasing and winsome tones are a far cry from the anguishing reality and stressful daily grind (pun intended) of most dentists. Many of the tales are in fact raw and disturbing yet are sanitized and become milquetoast pablum with no bite. And then there are those imaginary and over-the-top dental volumes written by non dentists who think they are so funny. I think not. So I thought it was high time to give an unvarnished and realistic review of the world of dentistry from my unique prosthodontic perspective while channeling my love of juxtapositional irony, twisted comedy and sarcasm. This is not my first bout in the squared circle of the writing realm. Some readers may have already indulged in my previous literary offerings and hopefully found them enjoyable. Although loosely based on my recollections of actual events, this book is "technically" fictional. It is a book of humor and should be taken as such. There is no malicious intent; the only intent is to entertain!

Dr. I. Mayputz

Foreword

For those entering the dental field, this book of "humor" will hopefully provide valuable insights into the *crazy* events that await you in your future career. You will quickly realize that working with dentists means you should have earned a psychology degree rather than a dental hygiene certificate! Each dentist has her/his own eclectic and eccentric personality and definition of perfection. Those unique characteristics can bring joy or doom to already hectic and chaotic days. Combine that with the unrealistically demanding patients and soon enough the Talking Heads tune *Road To Nowhere* roars through your head.

In time you will comprehend that you have created your own hamster wheel and may become frustrated by the continuous grind of dentistry. You also may become numb to the disturbing events that no dental staff member or patient should bear witness to. From the alcoholic dentist who shakes and drinks mouthwash throughout the day to keep his *buzz* going to the patient who runs screaming out of the office after a stab wound to the neck, the "fun" never ends.

No doubt at some point you will come to the awkward and uncomfortable conclusion that only HUMOR can truly

help you cope with the dental environment. What Dr. I. Mayputz has given the reader is a glimpse of a fictionalized playbook for the strangeness that may occur and to keep one's dental career in comedic perspective, regardless of the unpredictable shitshow happening around you.

P., RDH

TABLE OF CONTENTS

	Introduction	xii
1.	"Someone Stole My Choppers!"	3
2.	Teeth on the Cheap	6
3.	The Finisher	9
4.	Promising Beginnings?	13
5.	The Tooth from Hell	22
6.	God's Will?	28
7.	The Two-Timer	34
8.	Acronyms	37
9.	Diminishing Returns	49
10.	Gruesome Twosome	52
11.	Drug Me!	56
12.	Russian Teeth	61
13.	Make Me Over	68
14.	Marketing 101	75
15.	Bite Me	86
16.	Pre-Holiday Crush	92
17.	Crazy is as Crazy Does	99
18.	"I Don't Want a Damn X-ray!"	107
19.	I'm Dying	112
20.	Bad News	115
21.	Staying Ahead of the Curve?	123
22.	Confessions	130

23.	The Schedule	136
24.	Doggonit	141
25.	Crimes and Punishments	144
26.	Beware the Old Bag	156
27.	Kitty's Plaything	160
28.	Fighting Entropy	162
29.	Nice Guys Finish Last	165
30.	Back to Back	169
31.	"It Didn't Hurt Until You Touched It!"	179
32.	Sugar Daddy Dentistry	184
33.	Bridge Over Troubled Payment	191
34.	The Bad Penny	195
35.	Defensive Driving	198
36.	The Blame Game	203
37.	Continuing Education?	207
38.	"Herodontics"	217
39.	Who's in Charge Here?	221
40.	Same as it Ever Was	227
	Disclaimer	235
	Last Words	237
	About the Author	242

Introduction

Most dentists (excluding the ones only in it for the money) are a motley crew of somewhat naïve, frequently frustrated and serious perfectionists expecting gratitude and adequate monetary compensation from an indifferent and imperfect, yet demanding public. "Aggravation Saturation" is my coined catchphrase and aptly applies to the dental field in spades. Dentistry is not easy for the doctor and staff to execute or for the patient to receive. The daily dental shitshow can become a labor of hate and despondency for all concerned. Thusly, having even a smidgeon of humor can go a long way when trying to stay in the lane of the often inane and insane oral-healing world.

This book is about a slightly fictionalized account of chronologically selected slices from my lengthy career as a dental specialist. Embellishments of strange happenings were unnecessary because human foibles ran rampant. However, most names and places have been altered so as not to embarrass the guilty, berserk, bizarre, and downright scurvy. The yarns are what they are without color enhancement or pretrial publicity. The stories are retold in a series of vignettes which best captured my mood at the time. Who knew that dentistry could be so "funny?" Who knew, indeed? But is it ultimately a satisfying and

rewarding profession as well? I will let YOU be the judge and answer that last question. In the meantime, sit back, relax and at least snicker at my "pain." Hopefully you will find the tales within the following pages to be humorous and you will laugh along with me. Maybe at me, as well. And the jury is still out as to whether I would have done it all over again!

Enjoy.

Dr. I. Mayputz

WELCOME TO THE TOP 40
GREATEST HITS….
TO MY DENTAL PSYCHE!

1

"Someone Stole My Choppers!"

It was most likely the best set of upper and lower dentures I had made to date, and now I had to remake them! But why? Here is what transpired: I was a first-year prosthodontic resident at arguably the finest program in the nation at the time, at the Veteran's Administration hospital in the same city from whence I had graduated dental school. My master's degree specialization involved restorative and prosthetic dentistry such as the fabrication of dentures, crowns, implant-crowns, etc. Furthermore, I recently had not only restored that edentulous veteran's mouth to proper form and function but also used the photographs from the multiple steps involved as a case presentation to the dental chief of service, the prosthodontic director, and to my fellow prostho residents. It was all in the name of higher dental education and deemed necessary as part of our training. I was complimented all around by the higher-ups and my peers and, reveled in momentary satisfaction on a job well done. So why was that same veteran back in my schedule a week after the insertion of his "brilliant" dentures? Maybe it was for an adjustment, to relieve normal sore spots that frequently occur after delivery of new prostheses? That was probably it. I got my gold-colored denture lab bur ready for action as I affixed it into my slow-speed handpiece. A little drilling and polishing here and there and he would be good to go, I cavalierly thought. And then Joan C., my often MIA assistant, ushered him into my room. He appeared grim and didn't greet me with a toothy grin. "Some dumb fuck stole my choppers, Doc.," the grizzled old chopper pilot spewed out. What? Was he just making an inappropriate Asian funny, ie., Sum Dum Fuk? However, his sour disposition said otherwise, and he looked deadly serious. "How did it happen?" I incredulously queried him. "Well, after washing my plates I laid them down on the countertop and turned toward the urinal to take a piss. When I was done, I looked back and they were gone," he said. "Where did this happen, at your house?" I inquired. "No, right here on the first floor of the VA, dammit; in the men's room," he stammered, looking crestfallen and apologetic. Now, did an opportunistic vet really nick his teeth in hopes they would fit him? Was it the same as stealing someone's glasses in hopes the prescription matched yours? Come on. Was he a victim of a sophisticated bathroom heist? Was that shitter on the first floor a known clip joint? Or was he fibbing and perhaps sold his pearly whites to a gullible dumbbell instead? I did not know quite how to react and decided to take a quick jaunt to the VA Chief of Dentistry's office for some guidance. It was only down the hall in our dental service. "What's doing, Mayputz?" Dr. B. asked me in a flaccid, deadpan voice. After excitedly explaining the messed-up situation Dr. B. looked rather annoyed and flatly stated, "So, make him another pair. Why are you bothering me with such nonsense? Jesus fuckin' Christ. If he wants dentures, give him dentures!" But I had to ask his permission because Murphy's Law dictated that if I had not and went ahead with making the man a new set of teeth, the Chief would have gone ballistic and blasted me out of the dental clinic! You know how it goes; sometimes you just can't win. I reentered my operatory and proceeded to start the process of making new choppers, much to the delight of the formerly fierce aviator who had "lost" his. However, the new dentures somehow did not match the old ones I had made. The veteran was happy to have teeth again, but I was somewhat irritated at my inability to replicate all those subtle nuances that had made the first ones so "great." It was the little things that only a dentist would notice. Oh, well, I had done the best I could, and I never heard from that Vietnam vet again. I guess my second attempt wasn't too shabby after all.

2

Teeth on the Cheap

I was gainfully employed as a first-year prosthodontic dental resident at a well-known VA hospital, in the same large metropolis where I had earlier completed my dental school education. My pharmacist wife, infant daughter and I were living in a relatively close-by borough, but even that nearness necessitated me taking two buses, multiple subway trains and a long walk, in order to get to my workplace. It was an anxiety-filled and exhausting *schlep* each morning and evening but I knew it would end…. eventually. For those of you who never experienced PACKED city buses with unwashed, "crazy" folks onboard, urine-soaked, underground subways PACKED with wall-to-wall people, and "obvious" street muggers on the prowl for "pigeons," you really missed out! The early '80s were dangerous times in large cities with mine being one of the nation's leaders of *thug life* (the same as it is now). Anyway, it was one of those rainy, miserable mornings when, as I was hoofing it eastward on 23rd Street after exiting the 6th Avenue subway station, a trench-coat ensconced Black fellow rapidly approached me. At first glance he looked like one of those flashers that got their jollies by exposing themselves to women. I had slightly long hair at the time but with my manly physique did not resemble the fair sex in any way. So, what was his deal? He blocked my path and suddenly parted his long, wet raincoat. I was fully expecting to see dark nudity but instead was titillated by scores of watches, belts, earrings and trinkets that were fastened to the inside lining of his drab slicker. He mumbled a pre-rehearsed routine and also asked if I wanted to buy some loose joints as well. "I could *sens* it up all morning," as he put it (Sensimilla is a potent form of marijuana that was popular at the time). It was all cash and carry, illegal, but he had it all. I'm sure if I had asked for a bologna sandwich, he probably could have produced one as well! I recalled a similar confrontation I had years ago with a Black fellow from whom I ended up buying a knock-off Rolex watch for thirty-five dollars. I guessed these guys canvassed the city accosting tourists and hapless White suckers and losers like me in hopes of a quick sale. Anyway, I nodded NO to him and started to walk away but not before spying what I thought was dentures suspended next to the Mayor Koch bobblehead dolls near his left armpit. I stopped and motioned him back to me. He ran over and opened up his garments' flaps like a giant vulture and almost engulfed me with them. I don't know what the passersby thought of an umbrella-wielding, white-clothed, White boy having a tête-à-tête with a tall, nervous-looking Black gentlemen and I didn't care. Those were genuine false teeth hanging there! Are you kidding me? Five sets, in different sizes, with tiny holes in them for small wires to run through to affix them to the innards of his slimy overcoat. I laughed out loud as he asked me which ones I desired. As I convulsed with mirth, he told me that they were fifty bucks a pair and ready for chomping. After telling him I was a dentist and just curious, he grimaced, closed his "shop" and proceeded to illegally jaywalk across the street at a fast clip, continually on the hunt for paying customers. He had wasted precious time on me and had to stay one step ahead of the *Fuzz* while trying to make a few nickels peddling his shit as a "street solicitor." From where he procured those artificial teeth I do not know. Were they made in China, or Chinatown, or by a reputable local dental laboratory as a lucrative side hustle? I don't know. I kept on shaking my head as I approached my destination and marveled at the sheer *chutzpah* of some people.

3

The Finisher

The chief of the VA dental service was a short, stout, bearded, middle-aged prosthodontist and the head honcho of the highly coveted dental residency program I was enrolled in. Even though there was an actual prosthodontic director of our three-year specialty curriculum, the chief was the de facto leader of us five, prostho residents. And I couldn't say anything bad about him because, after all, it was he who had hired me. It was a great educational experience mainly because I was getting paid a decent salary while across the street at my former dental college; postgraduate students were paying big bucks in tuition to learn the same fare as me. Winning! However, near the end of my term at the VA hospital, the chief summoned me to his private office for an unscheduled powwow. Uh oh. With phony enthusiasm he feigned appreciation for all my years of hard work, blah, blah, blah…. but then launched into a back-handed compliment that threw me off-guard. He expressed concern that I had not worked on as many patients as my fellow residents had. However, before I could rebut his alleged and seemingly callous claims of laziness, he shushed me and continued: "You have evolved into a finisher, Mayputz. Unlike the others here, you finish what you start," he firmly stated. "You may not have done as many cases, but the ones you did never came back," he sardonically added. "Was that a good thing?" I thought to myself. What was he getting at? I began to tighten up and feel my temper rising. I had no beef with this guy; I had done everything as required. Why was he pulling my chain now, right when I was about to leave? Perhaps he wanted to get his last dental digs in? Maybe he never liked me that much in the first place? All those thoughts were bouncing around inside my pea brain as my anxiety level hit the roof. He then proceeded to give me unsolicited advice about my future. He emphatically declared that all a thriving private dental practice needed was five hundred active patients, in total, to be profitable. I must have had a strained and puzzled look on my sweaty brow because he continued. "All a dentist has to do is to recycle them. You don't necessarily need new blood, just milk the same ones over and over again." I had calmed down by then but didn't quite understand, and then he spelled it out for me: "You are a finisher and will never MAKE IT unless you become a milker," he slowly enunciated as if speaking to a four-year-old. "Work on your bedside manner to keep the patients, and then keep milking them forever!" he snorted. Again with the milk metaphors! Was that an insult because he knew I originally hailed from farm country in Upstate New York? However, I just sat there unmoving while staring at my brown loafers and thinking nasty thoughts about him. Nevertheless, finally it sunk in and I got his not-so-subtle drift. I tepidly thanked him at the time while still feeling slightly aggrieved. However, as I recently reflected on my three decades of prosthodontic dentistry, I thought about what he had said. I have always been surrounded by multitudes of arrogant "shoemakers" who busily cultivated the Gift of Gab instead of honing their dental skills, ones who had successfully convinced their unwitting patients into becoming ever-returning customers. Unfortunately, fillings turned into root canals, then into crowns, then extractions, bridgework, dentures and implants. It was a graduation of sorts for the hapless patients involved. The same gullible and ignorant clients were continually being milked for money while simultaneously being held on the hook with soothing syllables. Yet none of them were ever "finished," either by happenstance or by design. How do I know all this? I have seen many teeth that were hacked up by the "smooth talkers" in town and have had to bail out those dentists on numerous occasions, whenever they referred their abject failures to me. I generally dislike labels, but I'll take being called a finisher over a milker any day. And, yes, I did manage to scarf a few *shekels* from the hoi polloi during my lengthy dental career, whether continuously and gratuitously gabbing or not.

4

Promising Beginnings?

I had completed a prestigious three-year prosthodontic (prosthetic dentistry) residency program in 1989 and was highly recruited by a popular and "super-successful" older dentist in Upstate New York. I had the *cred* and he had the *crib*, AND the *bread*. What could go wrong? Plenty! Let me tell you: He had heard of me through a dental equipment salesman/broker who in turn had known about me from his own head-hunting sources. Although I had multiple lucrative opportunities to stay and practice in the city, I decided to move my wife and infant daughter to the Capital District area, close to where we originated from. Plus, this dentist really wanted me. It felt good to be wanted. And he promised me the world, or so it seemed. I was to be his associate and gradually take over the practice, in a time-honored and honorable transfer of power based on a handshake agreement between two dental equals. Ha! What a joke. What a naïve *putz* I was. I recalled that during our initial meeting he told me that he was close to retirement and that his previous, ungrateful associate dentist had surprisingly left after a seventeen-year stint with him. He further added that he rarely took a vacation and was well-respected in the community by patients and peers alike. Well, it turned out that at least some of that sentence was true. But I didn't care at the time. I would be paid fifty percent of collected monies minus the dental laboratory charges. It all sounded so generous, rosy and attainable. I was enamored by that very short, stout and engaging older dentist, one with tons of energy and tons of postgraduate degrees hanging on the walls of his office; he seemed to have it all. He had finished second in his dental school class and stated loudly that I was the *smart* heir apparent he had been searching for. I felt great and validated, and my ego soared. I was swimming with the idea of eventually having my own multi-million-dollar practice and raising my family in a favorable environment, coupled with fantastic public schools, etc. Things started out slowly, however, with Dr. E. only giving me some of his patients to work on. I had assumed that I would get half of his patient roster right off the bat, but it didn't happen. And when I confronted Dr. E. about his near retirement and "chronically" sore shoulder, he smiled coyly and said that he wanted me to build up my own patient base within his office. What? Why did he suddenly appear so greedy? He would be paying me fifty percent on my OWN patients? Was that fair? And how was I to get those paying customers? Advertising? No one knew of me just yet; I was the newbie face in town. And there was no written and signed contract between us, remember? I immediately phoned his previous dental associate, who had started his own practice in the next town over. He was the same piker who was continually badmouthed by Dr. E. That previous associate laughed his ass off when he took my call, called me an idiot and wished me good luck before slamming the receiver down, rudely hanging up on me while still cackling. I started to panic. What did I get myself into? So far I had only seen a handful of patients, had no assistant and was working with 1950s equipment. My fear of failure was supplanted by a fear of being in the wrong practice with the wrong set of ideals. Luckily my wife was working part-time as a pharmacist to keep us financially afloat while I wrestled with sleepless nights worrying if I had made the wrong decision. We could have stayed in the big city and I would already be making big bucks, and after only a few weeks of practice! But then a brand new male patient buoyed my sagging spirits and scant bank account. However, the seemingly sanguine initial consultation was by accident as I soon learned. The patient's socialite and well-connected wife had made the appointment and she wanted top "prosthodontic" treatment for her well-known, cardiologist husband. When the front office receptionist (Dr. E.'s sister) took the booking, she heard the word prosthodontist and assumed the patient's wife meant me. I mean, that was my official specialty. I did not realize that Dr. E. also fancied himself a prosthodontist, an oral surgeon, an orthodontist, a periodontist and other "dontists." Although only a B plus general dentist at best, his office was like a black hole. Once a patient entered, he/she stayed put and received treatment, even if it was mediocre. There were no referrals out of the office, except for impossibly complex situations that even specialists could not remedy. That's the kind of office it was. Anyhow, the shit hit the fan when Dr. E. found out that I was going to treat the esteemed physician and he wasn't. He berated his long tenured but clueless older sister up and down for making such a rookie mistake but relented in letting me treat the man. Both the wife and husband were delighted in meeting a real specialist in our basically boondocks location. I was just hoping that I could do the dentistry. My task was to replace an extensive lower front bridge whose porcelain had chipped off over the years and looked unsightly when the patient smiled. It was a piece of cake and well within my prosthodontic wheelhouse. I had done hundreds of these in my residency and produced another gem, much to the delight of the physician and his wife. They promised to tell everyone they knew about my comely demeanor and professional services. And Dr. E. facetiously trumpeted my success to the couple and to his office staff as well. I was beyond giddy. I got paid handsomely for my efforts and looked forward to more cases like that. Perhaps this gig was going to be alright? However, I never saw another patient like that again; Dr. E. made sure of it. After grinding away for six months making very little moola, I approached Dr. E. with a bevy of grievances. My patient load was not increasing, my personal expenses were mounting, and I was getting antsy about taking over the practice. Dr. E. looked up at me and said, "You've only been here a little while, you've got a lot to learn. And as far as buying the practice, you have no money. I should know because I pay you!" With that last remark he laughed long and hard as I cringed at the words. I subsequently found out that he was a selfish and workaholic dentist. He had had many businesses outside of dentistry fail: his car dealerships, real estate empire, steel factory ownership and building contractor-ship all went belly up over the years. Whether he was continuously paying off bushels full of debt or desperately wished to maintain his bourgeois lifestyle (he had two maids, a cook and full-time gardener in addition to a tall, blonde, trophy wife), I do not know. But he was constantly working. With nary a day off, and never a sick day or vacation, I quickly got the message that he not-so-subtly sent to me: He was NEVER going to leave or sell out. It was all a big, bogus scam to keep me in my place as his potential ace in the hole should things go south with his health. I was NOT a potential partner or owner in the very near future even if I had come up with the requisite money. Instead, I was a scut monkey at his beck and call. I ruminated on the fact that the previous associate lasted seventeen years in that same hellhole with probably the same pledges made to him. I was pissed and angry with myself. This is NOT how things were supposed to go. I was so stupid not to have done my due diligence about him beforehand. What a *schmuck* I was! I rather quickly made up my mind to leave and not be a part of this fraught, "owner-slave" relationship any longer. At first I didn't tell anyone in his office about my plans as I scoured the local area to find another job. I had heard substantiated stories of Dr. E. being a vindictive and remorseless thug besides being a money-grubbing asshole. As per the rumor mill, if he had found out I was looking for another dental position, he would try to block me and scuttle it. So, I took the initiative and went on offense. I deliberately announced my imminent leaving and used misinformation to keep one step ahead. I told the office staff in confidence (knowing they would tattle on me) that I was shuffling off to Kingston, N.Y., very shortly. Since I had no contractual obligation, I could leave at any time. Dr. E. pretended not to know but was probably secretly checking out every practice in the Ulster County area that had dental associateships to offer. Meanwhile, I looked slightly west and, after borrowing money from my old man for a down payment, bought into a large, insurance-based practice. The building was great, but the innards were dated, and the location was in a devastated city. However, the owner was making money and there was room for me. He was a *nebbishy* Jewish dentist who told me that he eventually wanted to leave the area. He would be taking along his lovely, non Jewish wife and two hybrid kids to join a kibbutz in Israel. Say, what? He also emphatically and enthusiastically stated that he had heard heavenly voices and knew what he had to do: to work as a Christian dentist near some confiscated olive groves in the West Bank. He didn't speak Hebrew, or even Yiddish! Whatever: I just rolled my eyes and didn't question anything! For all I knew he was a bit of a bullshitter and talked out of his hat, so to speak. However, for the present, I was part-owner of a practice and delighted to finally get my act in gear. Meanwhile I removed my diplomas from the previous wall of shame, packed some personal effects and walked out of Dr. E.'s office on a Monday morning with everyone, including him, staring at me. No one thought I was really serious about vacating the premises and Dr. E.'s pride took a hit as his parting words to me were: "You'll be sorry, Mayputz." I smiled and said nothing as I left. Our relationship had deteriorated to the point that we barely spoke to one another for the last half year of my employment there. Only later did he find out where I had landed and by that time it was too late to cause me any trouble. But what a rough beginning it had been for me. It was an ignoble waste of a year, not to mention the paltry salary I formerly received. As a highly touted dental student and resident, I messed up badly and wanted to set things right as soon as possible. Fortunately, my wife Hottie Blondie was solidly behind me as I took my new position at double the salary. Nevertheless, my story is unfortunately a common refrain among newly minted medical/dental personnel. This kind of unnecessary stressful and adversarial relationship is all too common and unnecessary because I also heard of stories where things did indeed work out. The benevolent selling "mentor" and eager "associate" worked things out amicably with the young dentist assuming the practice in a timely manner and with both sides winning. Mine was like a bad marriage that needed to be annulled in a goddamn hurry. And I got out, I had to. Oh, and Dr. E. just recently passed away as a widower at age eighty-six, still furiously working forty hours a week, and after a five decade stretch at that. He was the same jerk who tried to have me believe that he was ready to retire over thirty years ago. He had a bunch of associates over the years after me, all leaving for greener pastures after finally seeing the light and through all of his lies. And he worked on a Monday and died that evening. I heard that angry patients were trying to physically break down his office door on the following Tuesday morning because the frazzled staff was late getting to the office. Did patients eventually mourn his memory? I'm sure at least a few did. But I also got wind from a reliable source (one of his hygienists) who told me in confidence that many of his patients threatened to sue him and his estate for leaving them in the lurch. That's gratitude for you. Even in death patients still wanted a piece of him. No rest for the wicked! I sarcastically laughed at the news of that mean old miser's demise and even more so when the Dr. E. apologist, and then president of the local dental society, called me to solicit some kind and comforting words for the society newsletter in honor of Dr. E.'s "superb" fifty-year service to the community and his outstanding persona. Yeah, more like persona non grata in my book! I tried in vain to keep a straight face on my side of the blower and managed to contribute two words, "F... h.." and then slammed the phone down while still cackling out loud.

5

The Tooth from Hell

I had a few weeks of misery left at my present associateship before leaving for a dental practice I had recently bought into as a junior partner. Those weeks could not go by fast enough. But wait, first I had to treat an aching molar on a fortyish man who was stuck into my mostly empty daily schedule by the front office staff. I was a certified prosthodontist and as per my post graduate training, was best suited to treat complex restorative cases involving dentures, crowns, bridgework, implants, and cosmetics. Sure I could still do general dentistry and fill a cavity with the best of them, but I could do more. However, with this particular gentleman, I got less. He was a patient of record and felt comfortable being treated by the "ASSociate" dentist (me) and not by the "old man" himself. And it all started so routinely you know....banal pleasantries were exchanged, an x-ray of the offending tooth was taken and then - the bad news: "Mr. Hackelshmackle, your back lower molar (#18) is abscessed, and you need to have a root canal or an extraction done. A filling won't do," I said in my most authoritative doctor voice. My anxiety level was still under control as I delivered the verdict and was ready to refer the patient to my boss or to a local endodontist (root canal specialist). However, before I could utter another syllable, the patient insisted that I save his precious tooth and do something now because of the great pain he was in. And I remembered the advice that Dr. E. (the practice owner) had given me, namely, to do "something" for every patient at every appointment. Talking, evaluating, referring or prescribing medications were not good enough. Patients wanted treatment and value for their visits, not just examinations and diagnostic chitchat about their teeth. Oh, boy. As my temperature and temper started to rise, I tried to dentally reason with Mr. Hackelshmackle and valiantly pushed for a referral solution. "Can't YOU do it, Doc? It's killing me. You gotta do something." He was right, of course. I HAD to do something. And there was that word again – something. However, I should have prudently prescribed an antibiotic and possibly an opiate pain killer, or Motrin, and referred him to an endodontist. Instead, I proceeded to try to get him numbed-up, and then reviewed the exacting procedure in my mind. I knew how to skillfully do molar root canals although I had not done one since dental school. I had finished plenty of relatively easy single canal cases since graduating but not a three-rooted one found in the back of the mouth! Suffice it to say that what transpired on that day and for weeks hence was a nightmarish scenario for me and the patient. I never, ever should have listened to him and been swayed into performing treatment. But I was young, cocksure, and needed every cent I could get. However, everything that could have gone wrong did, starting with me struggling with the damn rubber dam placement and the failure of the local anesthesia to take hold. After using my best block technique and a short acting local anesthetic called Carbocaine, I repeatedly asked the patient if he was numb. "I'm all frozen Doc, bombs away," he cavalierly and positively babbled. So I started in, only to have Mr. Hackelshmackle almost jump into the ceiling tiles and practically knock the handpiece (drill) out of my hand. WTF? "I thought you said you were numb," I shakily asked, my heart pounding a mile a minute, sweat starting to bead-up on my brow, and losing more hair on my head with every passing moment. "Are you doing the right tooth, Doc?" he questioned, barely able to talk because of the generous anesthesia I had already administered and with that piece of rubber sheet in the way. It was just as I feared. He was all bluster but highly apprehensive and super sensitive. So I gave him a few more shots. But it didn't matter: he continually "felt" everything as I tentatively and carefully tried to drill again. A hypersensitive and anxious patient is often the worst experience a dentist can encounter, often compounded with the ever-present time crunch breathing down her/his neck. It was all so terribly frustrating and defeating. I was fast running out of tricks and I had not even begun to do the arduous root canal therapy. After an hour of mostly futile starts and stops, I had to stop. With his head constantly moving about due to supposed discomfort I had managed to just accomplish the opening hole through the enamel. Even that was a big deal. I put him on an antibiotic and once again gave him the option to see an endodontic specialist. He grinned and said, "Why? You did great Doc; that was the best root canal I ever had." When I told him I had barely started he was shocked but agreed to come back again to "finish" it, because it was cheaper to do so in our office. However, I was exhausted mentally and physically. This was not how a root canal was supposed to go. Now, most molar endodontic procedures in the '80s took between three and four visits. Nowadays they can be done in one or two sessions with the futuristic and advanced three-dimensional cleansing and obturation techniques available. Without boring you non dental readers, suffice it to say that it took me eight visits with immense, unbearable stress and trepidation on both the patient's and my part. Mr. Hackelshmackle's lack of cooperation and my lack of an assistant greatly exacerbated his and my misfortune. I'm surprised he kept coming back; however, progress was being made, albeit in drips and drabs. He was no longer in pain by the fourth appointment, so that was a good thing. And when I successfully completed the therapy and clutched the final x-ray film in my hand as proof of a job well done, he finally exhaled and relaxed in the chair. I was still a bundle of nerves as I correctly closed the access hole in that darn tooth with cotton and a composite filling, and then dismissed him to the front desk to pay up. But eight visits instead of four had lost me money. That was not the way to practice or earn a living. Either I had to screen patients better or I had to get better, or both. Maybe it was an aberration and would never happen again? Well, it never did because I made sure of it. I never did a molar root canal again, no matter the begging or cajoling from my future patients. There were specialists for that kind of work and I stuck to prosthetic dentistry, as I should have. However, I made an exception and did one on my father recently and it was a piece of cake. It was my first molar root canal in over thirty years, and it couldn't have gone smoother. Two visits, no squirming on my part or pop's, and it was uneventfully completed. No problem. Perhaps Mr. Hackelshmackle and his darn tooth had been the guilty parties all along and unwittingly soured me on future molar endodontics? Probably because I still remember the lyrics and poignancy of that 1975 hit single from rocker Ian Hunter, *Once Bitten Twice Shy* (and no, Great White did not write it but successfully covered it in 1989, for all of you know-it-all and wannabe heavy metal, head bangers out there)!

6

God's Will?

I had successfully extracted myself from a dead-end and one-sided dental associateship position with a jerk of a dentist and bought into a large practice in a skeevy part of a city. According to the contract signed I was now a legitimate ten percent owner. This time things were in writing and hopefully would protect MY interests as well. The location of the office was decent, with plenty of parking and on a busy street. However, the surrounding area was a bit depressed and most of the patients came from outside the immediate locale. But it didn't matter to me where the money came from. I was just elated to finally get my foot in the proverbial dental door and start making my mark in the world of dentistry. I was young and enthusiastic, had a pharmacist wife and two young children, and needed to get my act in gear to be the provider they deserved. All I had to do now was get along with the owner and slowly navigate the often-treacherous waters to full partnership and possibly future ownership. And I didn't care what kind of dentistry I would be performing; hopefully it would be heavily restorative in nature, however. Even though a certified prosthodontist, I knew a multitude of similarly trained peers who basically did general dentistry to pay the bills with only a smattering of specialized cases thrown in here and there. I surmised that I too would embrace that model. Of all the dental specialties, prosthodontics has the most overlap with general dentistry. Yet the reverse is not true. Many general dentists think they are qualified prosthodontists and able to tackle tough restorative dentistry, unfortunately, that presumptuous paradigm is based on arrogant and faulty reasoning. Anyway, it was a heady and exciting time for me, and then I glimpsed that first handwritten biblical quote Scotch-taped to the dental lathe in the back of the office. It was displayed in a prominent position so any employee walking by could read it. When I questioned a few staff members, who were obviously brand new to me, they shook their heads and strode away without directly answering me. Did I join a religious cult without knowing it? Was the practice owner responsible for that religious gibberish? It had to be him. Who else could it be? But I thought the bearded and manly Dr. S. was a straight shooter, a decent dentist, and an all-around nice guy? Plus, he was Jewish. Only Orthodox Jews and their over-religiosity could explain his actions, yet he did not wear a yarmulke or dress in black, Orthodox-type clothing. So, what was really going on? Did he fool me into joining his practice under false pretenses? Did he in fact have diabolical plans for me that did not involve dentistry? I immediately confronted him in our shared private office. He was taken aback by my confrontational queries and explained in great detail that my coming to his dental practice was foreseen by God. What? He went on to say that he and his immediate family were Messianic Jews, or Jews for Jesus. He was a devout, speaking-in-tongues, evangelical Christian of a certain sect and not Hebrew in his religious convictions. His *shiksa* wife was also a Charismatic Christian believer and they both had prayed long and hard for me to come along and deliver them to the Promised Land for their true calling. What? At this point I had to sit down as I listened with my mouth slightly agape. Dr. S. further stated that the biblical sayings that he routinely posted around the office were for him as personal reminders of his ongoing piety and fealty to the Lord. Oh, boy, what did I get myself mixed up in? And then the real bombshell: "Izzy," he proclaimed in a deliberate and startlingly ominous voice, "You have been chosen by God to buy this dental practice so that I may do his bidding and go to Israel to convert people in the name of Jesus Christ." What? Was I part of a comedic sitcom called "The Holy Rollers Go to the Holy Land"? However, he was dead serious as I kept staring at his nervously twitching eyelids. Was this guy nuts or what? And whose God was he referring to? I didn't know. Fast forward a few weeks and I found out a few other things as well. Because his practice was basically an insurance mill, quality dentistry was often eschewed for the sake of expediency and a packed schedule. The insane volume of foot traffic mitigated the low fees charged and acceptance of many dental insurances as full payments for services rendered. I prided myself in being a relatively fast dentist without compromising excellence and spliced in quite nicely into the money-generating standard of the office. But I continually "heard" things about his personal brand of dentistry that were very unsettling. One incidence was of him indifferently "making" a crown fit over a tooth when it was in fact supposed to be inserted on the same tooth but in a different patient's mouth! You know, little things like that, which not only violated Christian moral values but more than a few dental/legal tenets. Was he maliciously unethical or was he a victim of circumstance because of his break-neck work pace? Who knows? Maybe that's what his Ivy League dental college (Penn) had taught him or maybe he learned those speedy dental hacks on his own? The longtime staff just shrugged whenever I reached out to them for answers. In addition, I was shocked to learn that he had never had a single malpractice suit brought against him in over twenty-five years of practice. Perhaps his God truly did favor him? It started to look that way. Fast forward a few more weeks and I found myself with an SBA loan for half of the practice purchase price with Dr. S. holding a seven year note for the rest. It was all happening so quickly, too quickly. I had anticipated a breaking-in period and yet, there I was, ready to take the reins of a large dental office as a well-trained but greenhorn dentist. Nevertheless, any butterflies I had dissipated as I put on my big boy pants and got ready to rumble. After all, I had been chomping at the bit to own my own practice, so…. this was it, sink or swim. And then I started to doggie paddle like mad as Dr. S.'s day of departure loomed. My financials were figured out, the staff liked me, and I already had a steady stream of paying patients lined up. All I had to do now was clean up Dr. S.'s desk, which resembled a beaver lodge with papers stacked up like interlocking sticks in a center point, and to show him the door. He and his family had their Israeli kibbutz in the West Bank all picked out and were more than eager to move. He had rapidly sold his house, furniture, cars and personal belongings and was all set to depart. He told me that he had extra bibles packed just in case of trouble and then he left; no party, no nothing. And just like that he was gone. The next day I solicited the help of his now redundant former dental assistant P., whom I did not fire. She watched in horror as I nonchalantly swept all the paperwork off his messy desk into seven large garbage bags, tied them up and threw them into the parking lot dumpster. "What if some of those were bills?" she lamented, with a worried look on her face. "Don't worry, I'll get second notices if they were indeed due," I laughed. And I was right. I was always a neatnik and stickler for order and quickly eliminated the wanton chaos of my new dental practice. The staff was relieved as were many patients, who privately praised me and almost universally uttered the same sentiment, namely: "Thank God it's you and not Dr. S. working in my mouth!" I guess it was no mystery as to the mysterious ways in which God works. And that is how I started private practice as an owner – through trial by fire, while under fire. As a small corollary to this story: Dr. S. only lasted a few months in Israel; I guess the "chosen people" in his newly built commune resented being converted to Christianity while getting their teeth mauled and while periodically being shelled by recently dispossessed and disgruntled Palestinians. He and his family subsequently moved back to the U.S. settling in the "Bible Belt" area of Ohio where he is probably still proselytizing to this day, in between speedily placed fillings of course.

7

The Two-Timer

It was early in my first practice as an official owner and already I had encountered multiple bizarre situations involving seemingly "normal" patients. And what's more, the hits kept right on coming. Nestor L. was a nutcase in point. Good old Nestor was a swarthy-looking, Latinx man in need of much restorative dentistry. You know, mainly fillings to fill the holes in his teeth; nothing unusual or out of the ordinary. He would always come in as scheduled, banter some banal small-talk and we would get started. However, after a slew of appointments I started to notice that either I was getting more dentistry accomplished per visit, and had forgotten to chart my progress, or he was getting some dental work done on the side. I frantically scoured my handwritten notes (before everything was on the computer) and at first wrote it off as an error of omission; perhaps I had failed to properly chart the dental work that I had completed. But then it happened again, and again. Just as I was about to begin drilling on an upper right first bicuspid, I noticed that it was already restored. What the hell? Was Nestor cheating on me? Was another dentist sticking his fingers in MY patient's oral cavity? Or was I the OTHER dentist? Finally, I confronted Nestor. He looked puzzled and politely stated, "You're the only dentist that I go to, Doctor Mayputz." Did he have a brain fart one day and walked into a similar looking dental office in another part of Skankectady and saw another dentist who resembled me? And then he kept right on patronizing that office? And that dentist never said a word or yelled at him? I stared at Nestor long and hard and didn't know whether to howl or scowl. What could I say? Could I get in any trouble? Maybe, but my records clearly showed the documented dental work that I had performed, and I couldn't be held responsible for anything else in his mouth. So, what did I do? Nothing. He paid his bills and showed up on time, which was better than many patients did. My assistant P. always chuckled warmly under her surgical face mask when we subsequently treated him but sometimes inappropriately guffawed out loud whenever I announced finding "foreign" dentistry in his cake hole. Was Nestor the same way at home? Perhaps he had two houses? Did he also have two wives, two sets of kids, etc., and yet calmly dismissed any normative and valid concerns as ludicrous? Was he that good of a straight-faced schemer and liar or just an embarrassed bonehead who couldn't get up the nerve to stop visiting either dental office? I'll never know the details because he eventually left my practice after I completed MY version of his needed dental therapy. Did he go back to the "other" dentist? I don't know and still don't know how I actually feel about the whole affair. Bizarro!

8

Acronyms

Oftentimes you have to be in the know, culturally hip, and with-it to understand and dispense the latest lettered abbreviations for phrases and expressions. LOL means laugh out loud, LMAO means laughing my ass off, BISH means Biden is still hidin', etc. And most of us are still aware of the oldie but goodies from yesteryear - PETA, the ASPCA and OPEC. But what about those four dastardly denizens from the world of medical acronyms: PPE, OSHA, HIPAA, and OPD? Although seemingly innocuous conglomerations of jumbled and harmless letters, the "stab in the back" effect they elicit can be excruciatingly stressful to doctors. Let me tell you about these invective alphabetic scourges, ones that can bring more than a tear to the eye of the beholder. Personal protective equipment, or PPE, is now physically commonplace and the common-sense attire donned prior to all dental treatments, but that was not always the case. As a dental student in the early eighties, I observed more than a few "wet-fingered" instructors initially balking at gloving and masking-up for fear of losing their "touch" when helping us treat clinic patients. We students were made to "dress up" for each and every patient encounter; that's all we knew. However, even in the midst of the Aids epidemic that was gripping our metropolis, certain old time dental professors resisted. I don't know what they did or did not wear in their private lairs throughout the city, but in our esteemed dental school I saw many bare and hairy hands immersed up to the wrists in saliva saturated mouths. Yuck. Therefore, the school, in its FINITE wisdom, issued a dental Fatwa whereby ALL employed dentists needed to be latex covered for everyone's protection or be fired. Well, reluctantly, the hand-condoms were rolled on and early Halloween masks were placed onto dour faces by the dentists and life went on. I mean brain surgeons could operate with rubber gloves on and yet my shaky-handed teachers were afraid of diminished dexterity when drilling a molar? Come on! However, PPE meant much more than that. Increased sterility practices and using plastic/latex disposable items gradually became the norm. Again, as lowly dental grunts, we had no say in the matters and accepted the increased vigilance and antibacterial/antiviral methods and were prepared to carry them forward into our future careers. Nevertheless, in my first professional foray as an associate dentist in a well-established practice only I, and not the owner, wore protective accoutrements and practiced sterile methodology and meticulous hygiene. His old-fashioned habits were hard to break, I guessed. I said nothing to him, but he should have known better. However, by the early '90s, when I was the new owner of a huge office, I continued my learned ways and assumed most modern dentists did as well. But au contraire, my assumption was incorrect! And then it hit – a joint and mandatory proclamation from the American Dental Association, the local dental societies and the state education department, namely, that all dentists were now required by law to ensconce themselves with gowns, masks and gloves during patient therapy. And new requirements were issued for the proper implementation of a multitude of disposable items. I chuckled heartily because I was already ahead of the curve, or so I mistakenly thought. What I didn't know was that as the demand for the suddenly mandatory supplies skyrocketed, the prices would rise astronomically as well. A box of gloves went from costing five bucks to twenty, if you could get any at all! At least all dentists were finally on board and I optimistically thought the clamor would simmer down as prices fell and supplies increased. But they did not at first and to add to the mounting frustration of dentists, all the before mentioned governmental dental entities unexpectedly made public service announcements touting the new and INEXPENSIVE equipment that should now be available in all offices at no extra charge to patients. What? I was livid, as were other dentists. The formerly cheap gloves, masks, plastic suction tubes, air/water syringe tips, gowns, bibs, face shields, etc., did not cost pennies on the dollar as dismissively squawked about by the powers that be but now dug deeply into the bottom lines of we bottom feeders in the trenches. Sure we all wanted to be "sterile" and compliant but who was going to pay for all these pricy, disposable products? Patients were privy to the same advertisements as us and thought that dentists would and could easily absorb the extra costs because we were perceived as wealthy charlatans anyway. And dental insurance companies did not reimburse us for all the mandated props either, citing that we had to absorb it. But I resented being an Absorbine Junior and taking it on the skin! Some offices incorporated the special fees into their overall charges but not insurance-based offices like mine. What I did was add on a small cash surcharge per visit to help defray the added overhead expenditures. And what ensued? Hordes of my patients were stunned that their insurance companies did not pick up the additional, miniscule fees and most refused to hand over the added ten-spot per treatment. That led to office arguments and bad feelings galore, all because of the lies perpetuated by OUR feckless dental organizations. Instead of helping us by properly educating patients and guaranteeing adequate equipment at reasonable rates, we instead had expensive new rules foisted on us, all in the name of prudent "government policy." Nevertheless, the initial bitterness of dentists waned as the '90s slowly dissipated and more latex was harvested in Malaysia and Indonesia. However, we should not have been treated that way in the first place. But no one cared and in the end most of us ate the elevated price gouges and stopped payments on our Benzes, at least for a while (I actually owned a '96 Honda Civic at the time, just sayin'). As the PPE wars diminished and things quieted down, another acrimonious acronym reared its ugly head. Yes, the federal occupational health and safety administration (OSHA) and its state tentacles picked the late '90s as the time to finally crack down on "derelict" dental offices once and for all. I mean we had it coming, didn't we? Poorly articulated office fire escape policies, unwashed floors, bad sterilization techniques, hazardous waste just lying around, soiled needles pricking disgruntled staff, general uncleanliness, etc. were just some of the scary dental scenes as outlined by OSHA; and ones that needed immediate remediation. Holy Mackerel, staff members and patients were NOT safe in most dental offices! Plus, the fines collected from the guilty parties would be a nice bonus for the government as well. Oh boy, not only were office personnel encouraged to snitch on their negligent bosses, but the Gestapo tactics used by OSHA officers were downright appalling and absurd. Unannounced visits, interrogations, and huge, capricious fines were levied right and left on practices that were not in compliance with the new and nebulous statutes. Many dentists, including me, became petrified and sought to adjust as quickly as possible. But just hold on there, Sherlock! Let's backtrack a bit first. Were all dental offices really in a perpetual state of disarray, sporting blood spattered walls coupled with prevailing unsavory and unsanitary conditions? Really? Well, maybe some were but I'm fairly positive not all. Anyway, after reading about the offices that were more than wrist-slapped, we rank-and-file drillers galvanized our resolves to comply, protect our employees, and get on with our dental lives. But how? OSHA cleverly did not release a bona fide code of conduct or specific policies for dentists to follow in order to keep offices compliant. As usual, it was another gotcha government trap. I was frantically reading and absorbing all the scuttlebutt at the time and the best OSHA could say was that each office had to maintain highly detailed records of all hazardous materials, have sharps containers and special red biohazard bags in each operatory, had to sterilize rooms between patient visits, had to have adequate PPE, had to have all sundries displayed on labeled shelves along with their hazardous potentials (MSDS sheets), had to have eye wash stations installed, had to spore test the autoclave daily, etc. Now, most of the new regulations made perfect sense; however, the minutes of required weekly staff meetings, documents of needle-stick injuries to employees, etc., and keeping comprehensive track of all of this was left up to the dentists. What? There was no uniform guidance or guidebook to which to refer to. I heard and read reliable stories whereby dentists were shaken down for thousands of dollars, not because of cobwebs in the corners, but because of inadequate records. No matter what the dentist showed or divulged to the OSHA "police" it was rejected, and fines were gleefully imposed. All that because of a vengeful former "whistleblower" employee or patient. It got to the point where we were all scared as hell. Was I in good standing? Would my office be inspected next? Those were unnecessarily nervous times; however, they too ended. After a few hundred articles were written in dental journals and after OSHA-beating specialty companies sprouted overnight, expounding on ways to be compliant, OSHA reluctantly backed off. The jig was up. Meanwhile, more than a few complaints from dentists had been lodged with local and state authorities about the merciless response from the federal government and its messianic zeal to oversee dental offices. The rules were ultimately relaxed, namely, a complaint was mailed first which could be rectified by a response letter without triggering an automatic office invasion. The penalties were lessened substantially and complaining parties were interviewed about the allegations before an office was potentially terrorized. And after all the resentment and frantic machinations by my fellow dentists, we could now breathe a collective sigh of relief. The last piece of the puzzle was affixing a large OSHA-mandated sign in the office which outlined the rights of employees and repercussions for the dentist for not adhering to them. No more brutal barging in to catch dentists in "the act," no more threatening phone calls, no more extraction of money for a nothing-burger. OSHA's intent of running roughshod on the medical/dental establishment was finally quelled. Thank goodness. HIPAA, the health insurance portability and accountability act of 1996, and not pronounced hippo, was yet another elephant in the dental room. Now what? Yet another invasive regulation to worry about? Why, yes, indeed! HIPAA is a complicated and confusing federal law that basically seeks to protect sensitive health information from being disclosed without prior written consent or knowledge on behalf of the patient. And with the additional Privacy Rule, patients can now control how their health information is used. I apologize if my broad definitions seem watered down; even I do not know the full scope of the statute. However, it was not the new law that buffaloed doctors, but the resultant cockamamie compliance with it. Let me explain: Offices, including mine, had all the right forms and patients dutifully filled them out. We were all on board, or were we? It was because of the new and heightened level of intra-office secrecy that led to big problems. Staff could no longer leave charts exposed on the countertops for fear of patients reading other patients' names and surveying their private stuff. All paper charts had to be filed away and hidden from physical view, and the appointment book needed to be kept closed at all times. Staff could no longer gossip out loud about Mrs. Jones' bad tooth or Mr. Jones' list of surgeries and medications. Many dentists went so far as to soundproof their operatories and hang doors on them, all to contain any accidentally spilled verbiage which could be construed as a dereliction of duty by the practitioner. Whoa, Nellie! It became moronically stressful to work in a monastic and paranoid office environment, constantly whispering and not knowing what jargon was appropriate. And this was way before the politically correct and "cancel culture" kooks reared their "woke" heads! Savvy and smart-alecky patients would eyeball me and my staff just waiting for a slip-up. Some would joyfully reprimand us; some took us to task and threatened to report us to the state education department or OPD, the office of professional discipline. It seems funny now, but in 1997 the palpable daily office tension was real; no one wanted to screw up on purpose. I recall the first time I had to phone another dentist to discuss a referral of a patient after the new regulations became law. Could I even speak to him? Could I discuss the patient's medical and dental history over the phone? Could I talk to a staff member about that patient within earshot of other employees and patients or did we have to go into the parking lot outside? I mean the patient had signed ten sheets of HIPAA documents allowing me to do something or other in an emergency; was this one of those times? Would the other doctor report me? Although appearing silly now, those were valid concerns back then. With OSHA henchmen still lurking around, one never knew for sure if and when federal HIPAA "enforcers" would show up at your doorstep as well. Thankfully, multiple clarifications of the decree emerged through written articles in dental magazines and from continuing education seminars that featured knowledgeable governmental lawyers. Whew. Dentists had dodged another bullet, with most of us never purposely or egregiously violating the federal edict. But get this: I recently "heard" that the U.S. Department of Health and Human Services is proposing to relax some of HIPAA's Privacy Rule policies allowing for easier interactions between doctors and patients during emergency situations, etc. Really? Duh! It only took twenty-five goddamn years for HIPAA to start crawling back from the dark side! But I'll take it. And this leads us to the last acronym already briefly mentioned: OPD: the office of professional discipline. These are the three letters that doctors do NOT want to see linked together anywhere on their desks at any time! A letterhead with those conjoined initials on it is a most disturbing and frightening event for a practitioner. It's never good news. It means that a patient or third party (insurance company) filed an official complaint with that particular regulatory body and the doctor has to appear before an OPD commission and answer for it. And that's only the beginning. There is an upward chain of punishment from other state departments ultimately resulting in the removal of a license should exculpatory answers not be provided along the way. In other words, OPD is only the tip of the iceberg as far as getting into major league trouble. Of course, there are other avenues of redress for allegedly aggrieved patients such as a malpractice suit, small claims court, submitting a complaint to a local medical/dental society peer review committee to get money back, or just plain arguing with the practitioner to settle things. However, being reported to OPD usually indicates that an enraged patient wants to vindictively punish the doctor for a perceived slight. It is often less due to a technical/ethical/insurance problem than it is to a grave misunderstanding and a conflict of personalities between patient and doctor. Ce'st la vie. I have unfortunately been the victim of one such brush with OPD; the sordid story appears in this book. It was a deeply humiliating and unpleasant experience and though miraculously vindicated of the major charges, an extorted monetary fee had to be paid anyway because the three dental adjudicators (stooges) had to find me guilty of something – incomplete record-keeping. Give me a break. But that is how OPD justifies its existence, plus the punitive fines it generates ain't too shabby either! So there you have it, three medical/dental acronyms that can potentially bring much angst to doctors with the fourth, OPD, still remaining more than a phantom menace.

9

Diminishing Returns

The well-dressed and well-spoken senior gentleman had made himself comfortable in my dental chair as my assistant P. clipped on the blue bib and tucked it under his chin. He then pulled out his "newly made" full lower denture and simply asked me to adjust it. He had had it made somewhere else and for some reason did not, or could not, return there for follow-up care. Being a young, cocky dentist, full of piss and vinegar, I intoned in a swashbuckling manner that I could easily and effectively remedy his painful battle with sore spots. And then he could quickly be on his way. What a dope I was. Instead of carefully teasing out the truth from Mr. A. Conmann, like a fool I rushed headlong into trying to alleviate his dental malady. I checked his lower mouth and curiously did not detect the telltale signs indicative of a rubbing new denture. The patient then physically showed me where it hurt with his right index finger and I took his word for it. I mean, why else would he be here? If he said the plate was bothering him then it was bothering him, correct? Then he just sat there without saying another word as I got my acrylic adjusting bur whirring in the slow speed dental drill and started to nick off the supposedly offending spots on his denture that corresponded to the discomforting regions on his edentulous ridge. Well, as you might have already guessed, after at least thirty, free-of-charge, minor "shaving visits," he kept reappearing in my schedule to have more taken off that "offending piece of plastic," as he put it. Finally, I had enough and told him point blank that if I continued to "cut up" his artificial teeth, there wouldn't be anything left of it; it was already thinned out so much that at this point even a poorly trained dentist would have deemed it a massive failure. It resembled a narrow-bladed boomerang rather than a retentive oral appliance. It now fit like boots on a rooster! And all my intra-oral poking and prodding at his seemingly healthy lower jawbone revealed nothing unusual in the interim. What was going on here? What was I going to do? Then Mr. A. Conmann answered for me. "Doc, since you ruined my 'new' denture, how about making me another one at no charge?" he flatly and accusatorily stated. And there it was, the answer that had been hanging around the dental operatory all along, yet I had been too dumb to notice. I broke it so now I had to buy it! What a rube, what a dolt I was. He had hooked me like a hungry bass asshole, and we both knew it. He had intentionally wanted me to cripple his lower denture and then coerce or threaten me into fabricating him a new fixture. The oral prosthetic I had so diligently and judiciously adjusted was probably an old one that never fit correctly in the first place. He might even have had more choppers at home. And I'm not talking about souped-up Harley-Davidsons here! I had taken his initial word and like a stupe fell headfirst into his cunning trap. But instead of being outraged, because I could not prove any such salacious behavior on his part, I reluctantly swallowed my pride and made him a full lower denture at no cost. But I also harshly told him that I would only adjust it twice within a thirty-day period and then no more. He happily agreed and that was that. He did not show up for any adjustment visits after I had inserted the remade denture and I felt relieved. Nevertheless, I sadly tallied up the total of wasted time and money on that asshat and reflected on my loss of dental empathy in the process; it was most upsetting and disturbing. And I thought I was real smart; a smartass perhaps, but I had a long way to go before I could outsmart the many con artists out there.

10

Gruesome Twosome

No married couple appeared more physically and mentally disparate, or more dysfunctional, than that one did. Granted it was the second marriage for both, but, come on! Nancy R. was slightly portly and possessed that annoying, needling and overly loquacious personality. You know, the kind that just grates on you from the get-go. She was a new patient and had a mouthful of failing gold restorations, placed ages ago by her "incompetent and ancient" childhood dentist. At least that's how SHE described him. Her husband was a large and uncouth brute-of-a-man originally hailing from French-speaking Quebec province. He reminded me of a lumberjack straight from the backwoods and he spoke in very loud, simple syllables as if he had never attended school as a child. Nancy R. fancied herself to be a dignified and polite lady whereas he personified a roguish thug and purposely played up his eccentricities. He was a rough and tumble Canadian Canuck and damn proud of it. Nevertheless, they did not seem to be a good match as husband and wife, what with her constantly complaining about him and all. However, I guess love and sex were enough glue to keep those two

lovebirds together, eh? Anyway, her mouth was a
catastrophe, as was his. But his approach to treatment was
more straightforward, namely, to pull out all the "rotten"
ones as needed and replace them with "store-bought,"
partial dentures. In contrast, she wanted to save as many
teeth as possible, especially the gold ones which she had
paid a lot of money for. As I tentatively began her multi-
faceted and multi-stepped dental therapy, she just kept
yakking away. And the growing complaints about her
previous dental experiences invariably surfaced at every
subsequent appointment. Good gravy, I thought, her old
dentist must have been a real winner, a real Bozo. She
continually told me harrowing stories about that mean-
spirited, small town "tooth-puller" and the puny village she
had grown up in. Some of it was comical but mostly
vindictive diatribes on her part. But in the meantime, she
and I had a cordial and professional dental relationship,
and she valued my ability as a "Patch-O-Dontist." I did the
best I could repairing and refilling her numerous toothy
inadequacies instead of recapping or extracting blatantly
broken-down teeth. However, she was pain-free and happy
as I continued to patch up practically every tooth in her
head. Oh, I had documented everything including the
preferred course of treatment but kept conservatively
crawling along to satisfy her. As for her husband, who

would routinely regale me with stories of going to the great white north to help his "nearly feral" brother harvest potatoes while living in a shanty with Nancy, things were more forthright. He wanted plates, so I gave him plates! And his Francophile accented responses to me were patently the same: "Very good, Doc., very satisfied, very satisfied." He was definitely a man of few words and always answered me in those guttural and clipped sentences. Both he and his wife were just too much, and I was excited about completing their dental work and perhaps only seeing them in the future for touch-ups and hygiene exams. I was stoked at our mutual parting. However, as I was hopefully doing my last adjustment on his partial upper denture, Nancy R. strolled into the treatment operatory, greeted me, and then nonchalantly asked where I was from. I told her I was born in a large city in western New York State. Well, that placated her for a few seconds before her next query. "But did you grow up there as well?" she further quizzed me. "No, I grew up in a no-account, dinky and dusty farm town called Bumfuck, N.Y.," I said, as her eyes grew wide and mine narrowed. What did I say? Crap! Why were she and her husband laughing so hysterically? Well, it turned out that she was also from the very same Bumfuck, N.Y., and the maligned, gruff, old Dr. Smythe had been my family's dentist as well! I couldn't make this shit up if I tried. I had inadvertently opened the floodgates, crossed the boundary of patient-doctor interaction and became an unholy family member of theirs. Holy Moly, I swear I didn't do it on purpose. Anyhow, to make a short and effed-up story even shorter, they did not leave the practice as scheduled but continued to "bug" me for years with unnecessary appointments just to say hello and catch up with a *former* homeboy. Sheesh! Twice yearly hygiene visits were not good enough for them. Now granted, Nancy's husband was not from our mutual backwater settlement, but he had heard enough about it from her to make it his mentally adopted town. He politely pretended to be in on the gag and begged me to tell him tales about my upbringing while I was "adjusting" his perfectly made oral appliances. This was right after I had "worked" on Nancy to "fix" unbroken molars while also chatting and gossiping up a storm. What was wrong with them? What was wrong with me? Some patients become your friends, some become your enemies, some remain indifferent, and some end up being weirdly "different." At least I had gotten paid for all my mental trauma as I was befriending them against my will and while unintentionally crossing the line of dental professionalism.

11

Drug Me!

Herman M. was on the schedule as an emergency side-book that day. Oh, goodie, yet another late entry to the already heavily crisscrossed page which was part of the thick appointment book lying at the front desk (no computers back then). There was more pencil graphite than paper in that fateful ledger! Anyway, Herman M. was a disheveled disaster, as were his remaining teeth. I have seen many patients in painful distress and fully expected the young man in my chair to beg me for much needed dentistry because his examined mouth revealed a train wreck. "Let's start with some x-rays," I methodically stated. "Can't afford them Doc," he quietly said. "Ok, then how about just one for the teeth or tooth that bothers you the most?" I suggested. "Ok," he murmured, as he pointed to a bombed-out molar on his lower left side. While my assistant P. was developing the lone radiograph, I began the oral evaluation. Overall, he was suffering no obvious discomfort and my poking and prodding did not elicit any hurtful responses. He seemed to be disquieted but in no hurry for any dental treatment to be proposed or rendered. I reviewed the x-ray and even a freshman dental student would have recognized the badly decayed and infected tooth that needed to be extracted. But before I could give Herman M. my expert opinion or pass judgment on his oral cavity in general, he blurted out, "Give me some Percodan, Doc. That's all I need. I got no money today. I promise to come back and get all this fixed." I sat back in my dental stool and nodded knowingly. As a former druggist my extensive pharmaceutical background kicked in and I instantly realized poor Herman M. was probably addicted to opioids. It was unfortunate that he was using his destitute dentition as a pretense with which to wheedle out a narcotic prescription from me. "How about if I prescribe an antibiotic for you, instead," I offered. "I need somethin' for the pain, Doc. Tylenol and Motrin ain't cuttin' it," he replied looking more desperate by the minute. But I thought he didn't really have a raging toothache? Anyway, I prescribed Amoxicillin and Vicodin (similar to Percodan), Herman M. paid in cash, and the dental appointment was over. Now, whether he actually took the antibiotic I do not know. But another visit was scheduled for us to start addressing his dire dental needs. Fast forward a few weeks and there he was, right on time, as he plopped down in my dental chair. I slowly explained the possible treatments available from simple extractions to root canals and implant-affixed bridges. He looked puzzled, stuck a filthy finger into his mouth and pointed to the same molar as he had done previously. "It hurts, Doc.; write me up some of them SUCKERS again and we'll be square," he calmly intoned. "What about pulling that SUCKER and fixing the rest of your damaged teeth?" I sarcastically countered. And then it dawned on me. I was being played for a SUCKER, just as he had inadvertently revealed to me in his Freudian slip. It was deja-fuckin'-vue: Herman sitting in the same chair, pointing to the same tooth with the same dirty digit, and me about to comply with his wishes and authorize a New York State triplicate opioid prescription for him. But this wasn't the movie *Groundhog Day*! I got mad, stood up and told him NO. I said in no uncertain terms that either we were going to begin legitimate dental therapy or he could leave the office…. He left with nary a whimper or whisper uttered and I never saw him again. But what if I had complied? Then what? Would he have kept on milking me? And what if I had not been the only dentist taken in by Herman M.? Was he getting a boatload of illicit drugs from a farm of empathetic dental sheep and made the rounds to shear us at will? I'll never know the answers to those questions, but I was very angry that day and am not ashamed to admit it….Mr. Dundler was late middle-aged, always well-clothed, and a locally "respectable" used car dealer. He was admittedly high-strung and always under pressure. He was also very loquacious and quick-witted, and I presumed it was all part of his act as an aggressive salesman. His previous dentistry with me had been boringly routine although I always noticed, and noted, that he needed much more local anesthetic than my other patients did, and for similar procedures. I chalked it up to biologic variability, namely, no two humans are exactly alike. However, during one appointment for a deep cavity, and after five shots (two is usually the normal upper limit), he was still not getting numb and I began to worry. Try as I might I could barely begin the restorative process without him wincing in agony. What was going on here? Was I injecting him with water? I looked at my used anesthetic carpules and they seemed legit so what the hell was going on? I stopped the presses and apologetically dismissed him promising to try once more at a later date. Perhaps there was something physiologically metabolic going on or a sudden anxious state had befallen him? I did not know but seriously wondered, nonetheless. And during the ensuing visit, the same thing occurred, with the same unexplained outcome. Perhaps the internal anatomy of the tooth was messed up; I was really dumbfounded. The jittery patient also gave me pause as I sat back and tried to come up with dentally/medically logical answers. I never used epinephrine (adrenaline) for my injections, so I was confident that I did not cause the shaky patient demeanor. Was it his lively personality and normal dental apprehension that was getting in the way of dentistry? I did not know as I hit the brakes and holstered my drill. But then, in a moment of candor, Mr. Dundler revealed to me that perhaps he shouldn't have done so many lines that morning prior to our appointment? Now I got it. He was a closet cokehead and his entire nervous system was literally shot! Although appearing "normal," he was a cocaine-addled *boof* and it was reflected in my inability to properly locally anesthetize him. And I never did restore the tooth that needed a filling. Either out of embarrassment or lack of confidence in me, Mr. Dundler disappeared from my practice. It was too bad because we had a good rapport going and he never demanded drugs from me. I sincerely hope that both Herman M. and Mr. Dundler eventually sought and received beneficial treatment for their addictions. As a dentist, sometimes it is hard to spot deleterious addictive behavior even if it is right under your nose, and face mask.

12

Russian Teeth

Boris was an Estonian-born bronze artist and earth-moving, heavy equipment operator. He grew up in Soviet Siberia during the cold war and, literally, in the cold. Then he and his poor family emigrated to the Great Satan which instantly became the great savior, if you know what I mean. They settled in a small hamlet close to my folk's village and, since both parties were immigrants and of the same ethnic background, eventually "found" each other. However, whereas my aristocratic parents had emigrated from Europe after barely escaping the communist manifesto, Nazism and WWII, "newly enlightened" (Russian communism collapsed in 1991) and former Bolshevik Boris was fresh off the boat, so to speak. Although younger in age, he, his wife and offspring bonded with my parental units, who were elated to show the new arrivals the ropes of living in the United States as best they could. Boris began casting bronze statuettes and figurines for a Brooklyn-based, Orthodox Jewish art dealer and operating a rented backhoe on weekends to make ends meet. He purchased an old Buick, his "bottle-blond" and brassy wife was waitressing, and his two arrogant and always track suit-attired young boys were attending my old public high school. Things were looking up for them. But then it came to his teeth, darn it. And that's where I came in, darn it. Mom and dad cajoled me into coming in on a Saturday to treat their "special friend" and I reluctantly agreed. Somehow I sensed things would end up fucked up and I was proven right. Anyway, my office was two hours away, but they had assured Boris that I was the dental specialist to see, plus I would be delighted to do his dental work for free. Was I really happy with that arrangement? Nobody had asked me ahead of time. Oh, well. My parents drove him to my practice and I watched as they disembarked in the parking lot. They looked like three bundled up "immigrants." I sighed; sometimes you just can't take that old-worldness out of a person. Anyhow, Boris didn't appear to be a bad bloke as he shook my hand with a sweaty grip and tepidly sat down in the dental chair. And that's when I noticed strangeness about him. He seemed overly fearful for a seemingly virile, grown-ass man and was fidgety and twitchy. Was it the reputedly brutal Russian dentistry that had made him gum shy (pun intended) or was it something else? I didn't know and was slightly apprehensive as he gingerly opened up his Smirnoff-vodka and Marlboro cigarette-conditioned oral chimney and pointed to an upper front row of gold teeth.

He spoke in halting English, interspersed with fluent Estonian and Russian, and explained that while he was satisfied with the previous necessary dentistry, he no longer wished to look like a golden grilled Gangsta Rapper from the *hood*. His flashy yellow grin, while a sign of status and means in Siberia, was not the way he wished to appear when speaking to well-heeled and well-bred American customers in the art trade. I nodded, understanding him in all three languages spoken, and politely proposed a prosthodontic mini makeover. And then he started to shake. What the hell? My folks had not said anything about any personal peccadilloes he may have had, and his cursory health history was unremarkable. Was he just a nervous Norton or did he have Parkinson's, or both? I had come in on my day off and instead of being rewarded with a grateful and calm patient, had a demanding, moving target in front of me, one that needed at least eight new crowns! That was not an easy dental feat to accomplish on a "good" day and on a "good" patient, and Boris was most definitely not one. He was fast turning out to be a Russian bear, instead. And I had not yet begun to fight, as Revolutionary War hero John Paul Jones once proclaimed! I called my father into the treatment operatory and in an accusatory tone intimated that the patient was already knackered, and I had not even started. He was a mental and physical wreck; how could I do any sophisticated dental work when he was so uncooperative? Pop and Boris had a chinwag as I took five and spoke to my mother in the waiting room. I was pissed off and felt used and abused. I was a proud prosthodontist, yet boorish Boris made me feel incompetent and insecure. And I did not relish feeling like that. Here was a lowly, free-loading, redneck Russky who had managed to push all my buttons at once. Nevertheless, pop and he had a productive talk as I cooled off and all parties agreed to get something dentally done on that Saturday morning. Boris and I compromised. I would get him numb, he would stop acting so immaturely, and we would try to at least get four crown preparations accomplished. I'm not sure if the local anesthetic worked or not because the patient was gripping my chair arms with all his strength as I gingerly approached his still trembling mouth. I explained that I had to section off his old crowns, re-prepare the teeth underneath, take impressions, and make temporary crowns. All quite routine for me and for patients in the know. And he should have known because he already had that kind of work done before! And yet, he was beyond anxious and distraught as I began. I drilled into the upper front crown and promptly broke off my special, crown-cutting bur at the business end of the dental drill. I chucked it and inserted another one, and it fractured as well. Wtf? Stainless steel usually cuts through gold like a knife going through soft Land O'Lakes butter. What was going on here? I stopped and quizzed Boris with my eyes. He then sheepishly told me that his old crowns were in fact only gold-plated and not the real McCoy. As a bronze and metallurgy expert he then added that the base metal used for his caps was a chrome-cobalt conglomeration, one of the hardest alloys to saw through. Great, just fucking great. I was experienced in removing such tough crowns but in an agitated and spastic patient it would be a lengthy nightmare. And it was. After going through approximately twenty brand-new and expensive burs, and after two sweaty hours of hunching over a swaying mouth, I finally finished step one. But wait, the anesthetic had worn off and I had to give him more. At that point he needed a break and I dismissed him for a quick time-out. We BOTH needed it. My good-natured mom jokingly asked me how things were progressing as I removed my facemask and glasses. I just glared at her and said nothing. She got the hint and at that point probably realized that she should not have taken liberty and brought this kind of unwanted horror show upon her only son. However, it was too late for alibis and recriminations. After having a much needed and relaxing smoke outside, Boris and his reeking oral smokestack stepped back into my dental den. I also stepped up to the firing line and finally got 'er done. And it only took a total of three stress-filled hours instead of one. But, hey, he would get four brand new, shiny, white caps and I would get zilch. You know, what's fair is fair. After two weeks I saw him on a Saturday once more, this time to insert the newly made, all-porcelain and highly esthetic crowns. The appointment went uneventfully, with no shuddering or snide remarks from Boris. He loved his new cosmetic countenance and thanked me with an exquisitely made, foot-high, bronze casting of a molar tooth, secured to a metal base. I gratefully accepted the present as he smugly looked on. When I casually mentioned that his previous gyrations and beratement of me were unappreciated, he winced a bit but then immediately quipped that that's how many people behaved in the "old Stalinist country." According to his previous "culture," arguing, fighting, kissing and making up were not mutually exclusive. He further blabbed that Siberian dental visits were often fraught with tension and distrust which then led to a whole host of emotions being expressed by both patient and doctor. I guess I was just an American wussy and couldn't take it like a real man. But what was his excuse for all his cowardly bullshit? I shook my head while clutching my third-place bronze trophy and cringed upon overhearing my mom empathizing with Boris as they were departing, over the plight of his children's teeth. Thankfully, he never graced my office again, and neither did his dentally challenged offspring. I think that he was happy with only his front four incisors being finished and had also astutely figured out that I would not be able to handle mangled baby teeth on screaming adolescent *boyz* built in his same mold. Thank you, Boris.

13

Make Me Over!

I was firmly entrenched in my very own and very busy, large dental practice when the latest American craze hit. Yes, medical makeover mania started to sweep the nation in the late nineties and dentistry was part of that juggernaut. But it wasn't good enough to merely mention the miracles of bodily cosmetic enhancements through print media. No, TV shows started popping up right and left showcasing the quick and easy aesthetic surgical procedures that could be done, oftentimes in one day! Patients volunteered in droves to receive free, life-altering sculpting as part of the advertising gimmick. Parts and pieces were either removed or added to make the humdrum human form a Golden Proportioned work of art and ultimately more sexually appealing. It always comes down to sex, doesn't it? Anyway, it was a heady time with dentistry barely able to keep up. But it did and one-day complete dental therapies were now hawked as the standard of care, if a patient could afford it. And along with this ludicrous yet lucrative trend came newly deregulated yellow pages advertisements from physicians and dentists alike. Now all you had to do was let your fingers do the walking in the back of a telephone book. While perusing some of the outlandish ads, you could easily find the "right" doctor to stuff your breasts or give you paper-white, Hollywood Chicklets. Pricy full-page advertisements showcasing before and after photos of "satisfied" models graced those *yellowed* pages and even I threw my hat in that ring. Although my dinky ad proclaimed my expertise in prosthodontics and all things dentally cosmetic, I observed many surrounding notices as false propaganda. Based on my purportedly superior post dental school training, I was supposed to be the "expert" in town. However, certain dentists were blatantly stealing my thunder and getting away with it. I was incensed and jealous. But it was all legal, as long as they did not call themselves prosthodontists. The words expert and specialist could now be used with abandon to fool the populace. And a new terminology called Cosmetic Dentistry sprouted overnight. Was it a specialty I overlooked? Was it recognized by the American Dental Association? Was I a cosmetic dentist without knowing it? I mean we all learned how to bleach (whiten), apply composite resin to, and cap and veneer the front teeth in dental school, so what was so special now? Everything was happening too fast. I personally knew the local dentists well and most did NOT become aesthetic mavens overnight; ones who were able to promise AND deliver top notch dental results to a gullible and frantic public. Or could they? About this same time, the American Academy of Cosmetic Dentistry was launched as a legitimate and exclusive organization complete with a strenuous entrance exam to gain membership. But was it real? Did a dentist really have to belong in order to be qualified to enhance the smiles of wannabe sex-starlets? And then the coup de grâce: In addition to the recent flood of magnificently Photoshopped articles appearing in mainstream magazines to mesmerize the public and fellow dentists, written by nationally "famous" names in dentistry, a strange new phenomenon emerged. Dental "Institutes" started springing up all over the country promising a quick education for dentists, one that was superior to regular continuing education seminars. All of a sudden it seemed like everyone had a "school" to teach dentists something. For only thousands of dollars, and for a weekend or week's stay, a dentist would graduate with an "official" document of authenticity and could now be considered a "specialist" in cosmetics and other dental fields. Were those "institutes" regulated? Were they legal? Could I start one in my garage, shed or basement? Perhaps? It seemed as though publishing a few stories in dental journals, a slick color brochure highlighting supposedly superior skills, and a good sales pitch was all it took to become a "professor" and hook some dental suckers. What about my three-year prosthodontic degree? Was it worth anything anymore if a *Joe Schmoe* dentist could leave on a Friday, attend the smarmy Spanky Institute in Florida, come back on Sunday, and be just as trained up as me? Wow, my head was hurting from the absurdity of it all. And were all those newly learned general dentists really up to snuff? Were THEY the ones I should aspire to? Holy Moly, it was suddenly a brave new world and I felt left out. But most importantly, were patients beating a path to their respective doors in a goddamn hurry, plunking down mucho moola and then leaving with grins resembling Julia Roberts'? Or did they end up looking more like Julia Childs? I can give you no satisfactory answers to any of the above rhetorical questions I asked. Suffice it to say that some dentists, including me, did see a huge interest in and a temporary bump in patient load based on that aesthetic fad du jour as it swept the nation. But whether patients received a higher level of treatment expertise from the "institute-educated" and Cosmetic Organization-belonging ones as compared to "regular" dentists is debatable. However, the many stories of mostly female patients that bit on that manic movement are cautionary tales to this day. I too had a few "hot" babes come in, with the liposuction, plumped lips, enhanced cheekbones and tits and asses already "done," who implored me to do "something" about their smiles. It was often the last piece of the puzzle, to complete the Barbie Doll fantasy-look. It was all so hurried and desperate as if there was a time-limited mating game going on for the best and prettiest. Oftentimes these patients left my practice because I could not accomplish all their wishes in a few hours like they had witnessed on TV, or I got too technical when trying to realistically describe the complicated process. I'm sure most went down the street to have their wishes fulfilled, to the typical dentist with a two-page yellow pages ad and a multitude of newly acquired "institute" sheepskins hanging in her/his waiting room. I also heard from reliable rumors that lots of the hurry-up cosmetic dentistry and medical procedures ended up failing, both in my area and on those too-good-to-be-true, TV makeover shows. Sure, things lasted for the immediate euphoric photo shoot, and then one boob started to sag while two front veneers popped out and then three root canals got reinfected. You can imagine how it went. Stupid, super-rushed medicine and dentistry rarely works out well except for the practitioner, especially if she/he charged an exorbitant fee and if a hold-harmless contract was signed between the parties alleviating the doctor from any future liability based on the work done. It was a crazy time and I hope at least some of the patients got their money's worth. And, hopefully, most of their busts are still in place! As far as the original dental "institutes" go, most are still around, as are even more ridiculous dental organizations touting the benefits of membership. I never joined those select clubs or spent a week at the Noss Rash, Havid Dornbrook or EL-VI "boot camps" to learn *advanced* dentistry that I already knew. As an aside, I wrote a scathing but basically tongue-in-cheek opinion piece in my local dental society magazine not long after the "make-over" brouhaha had faded. I sarcastically pointed out that perhaps people in our suburban/rural neck of the woods never chose to patronize us in droves because they were always more in love with their ATVs than TVs. Maybe our *home gurls* and *boyz* were less influenced by the media storm than everyone thought. The entire rage had appeared to be a West Coast and East Coast kind of thing, with folks in the middle and mountains not really buying into the beautification project, so to speak. And being fickle humans, perhaps appearing like that toothy and well-endowed Marie Osmond was no longer in vogue? Oh, brother, was I roundly criticized for my acerbic yet poignant report. Dentists I did not know came out of the woodwork to rebuke me in subsequent issues of the journal. Obviously bereft of funny bones, the nasty and vile blowback from certain straitlaced and pompous pricks belittled my dental acumen and sought to set the record straight: that cosmetic dentistry and plastic surgery were STILL alive and well in our boondocks region and I should shut the fuck up, lest I put a hex on any lingering "business!" Boy did I touch a superstitious and sensitive nerve. Wow, did potential patients read our journal and could my succinct diatribe rattle them? I think not. But I think I rattled a few dental cages, nonetheless. Fast forward to the present: I continue to sit in the back row during continuing education conferences and silently snicker while viewing the presentations, especially those involving the wholesale placement of white-colored, toothy falsies in ladies with size DD falsies. And I continue to periodically write twisted and sardonic op-eds that are surprisingly published in local dental journals, often critiquing the state of dentistry. I do it just to annoy and wind up my fellow highbrow dental brethren. Why not? I'm an old dentist now, what do I care? It's not as if most of those cut-throats referred any patients to me over the years anyway, so, screw them!

14

Marketing 101

Most financially disabled (poor) dentists profess to love dentistry and to that end invariably complain to all within earshot: that if they could only stick to drilling and filling, without the pedestrian and lowbrow money-collecting aspects of the practice, they would be successful and happy campers. Firstly, you can't run a solo or group proprietorship without making a profit at some point, and, secondly, what a load of self-effacing horse doodoo! Perhaps those miserable dentists have no money because they suck at dentistry and offer dental altruism as an excuse? Or is there more to it than that? Perhaps monetary management skills and science know-how don't often blend together within one person? Maybe some dentists really are cut out for the drilling but not the billing? Maybe so. Nevertheless, I love the business side as much as the clinical aspects of dentistry. However, it's the inhumane humans and unforeseen daily rigors that have ostensibly worn me out after a long bout in the dental ring. While in pharmacy college I took a useless course called Pharmacy Marketing, which taught me absolutely nothing. Of course, I was stoned much of the time during that class so perhaps the bootlickers around me did learn something, just not me. In dental school, we had a few quasi, marketing-type programs which did not apply to the real world. They looked great on paper but were in fact crap as I later found out. And this time I wasn't HIGH when I took those classes! I graduated to the adult world of dentistry not really knowing how to profitably run a fully staffed company and to deal with the multitude of fiscal responsibilities that it entailed. But I had enough smarts to realize that I had to get live bodies in the door who paid me; that was the bottom line. Affixing fees, dealing with dental insurance plans and other challenges such as paying taxes were secondary to the basic principle of first getting patients into the practice. However, how do you do that? That's where the title of this vignette comes in. To me, marketing was simply about advertising your wares, often subliminally and subtly, to get patients into your dental chair and then extracting a fair fee from them for services rendered. I know that marketing majors may take umbrage at my reduction of a four-year college degree into one simplistic sentence, but as a profit-minded health professional that's what it meant to me at the time, and I was mostly wrong! I had bought a very busy, insurance-driven dental practice where constant running around by my staff and me was the norm. The previous owner had never stopped to measure any logistical or monetary metrics of the business. It was busy, busy, busy, all of the time, with tons of patients coming in because of our dental insurance affiliations. Staff members never sought to hone their communication skills or to check up on the accounts receivables because there were no reasons to. Money kept pouring in like manna from heaven due to the sheer volume of patient traffic. If my heavily penciled appointment book (no computers back then) was booked solid for two months then "things" were normal and I was supposedly raking in the dough. However, after a slight recession hit in the early nineties my bottom line took a dive and I began to panic. After a few sleepless nights thinking about the situation, I finally realized that the main reason patients patronized us was because we took their dental insurances in full, or at least as partial payments toward the fees charged. It wasn't my engaging personality, deodorant type or winsome smile that brought them in. No, it was purely financial and if more of those TYPES stopped visiting us, we would be in real trouble. And when I finally sat down with my office manager (and I use that title loosely) to review the outstanding receivables I was horrified at the numbers. Thousands of indebted patients were grossly in arrears to us, yet our office policies were woefully delinquent in collecting the sums that were overdue. Some outstanding balances were over twenty years old. It seemed as though most people just flashed their insurance cards at my front desk ladies upon completion of treatment and pranced out of the office. The front desk minions were trained not to pursue any additional owed payments and the patients were trained not to come up with any cash! Most customers never had any intentions of squaring up, yet no one cared because new insurance money had constantly been flowing in the pipeline to keep the office in the black. Even I realized that this was no way to run a business as my office manager balked at me in surprise. After I expressed shock at how things were being run, she became shocked at my heated belligerence and threatened to quit on the spot. I persuaded her not to and explained that we had to reboot the office protocols of how to "secure and retain" patients and how to properly "charge and secure" income, and not just from the dental insurance companies. We needed a strategic overhaul of everything, and I meant everything! She wailed that she was way too old to change (she was decades older than me) and tried to explain that that's how things were always done. I was desperate and didn't listen to her howling in protest because I knew that if I didn't start the process of rebuilding, revitalization and rejuvenation, my office would slowly start to die. And that's where my marketing instincts, or lack thereof, kicked in. First and foremost was to have new and existing patients want to make appointments with us, and not only because of our allegiance with their insurances. But how do you do that? How do you conquer the cemented mindsets of both clients and staff? I didn't quite know and had to start at the very beginning and not be shortsighted. But I have to confess that I had a little help in my initial marketing endeavors. My private office desk was usually littered with the latest dental rags that I received free of charge. And wouldn't you know it, after that mini recession had hit our nation, many "dental gurus" started writing about how to survive and thrive. And that's just what I wanted to read about. And read and learn I did! Firstly, I already had a beautiful looking building on a busy main throughfare, although in a skanky city. However, I had no illuminated signage by the road proclaiming my presence night and day like the dental offices across the street did. So that was the first step: get a brand name logo and sign to make my office unique and easily recognizable. Ha: Easier said than done. Part one was easy but not part two. Mayputz Dental was the name emblazoned into the middle of a large, white, winking and smiling tooth caricature. I had that symbol, along with the office address and phone number, imprinted onto lime-green juice bottles, toothbrushes, hot-pink pens, ice scrapers, toys and other giveaway freebies and displayed them all along the main office counter for patients to take. It was a colored cornucopia of Chinese-made, knickknacks and knockoffs. But take them they did. Afterall, they were no-charge goodies! Getting a sign posted outside the office building proved to be problematic, however. After hiring an expensive lawyer to plead my case and after three lengthy presentations in front of the town zoning board, I was summarily denied a small, free-standing sign next to the road. When I vehemently protested that my surrounding hokey dental competitors all had huge lawns signs, I was soundly rebuked and told that I had a professional structure and not a house practice. If I desired posting any sort of billboard it would have to be affixed to my building. Alrighty then, let the games begin! I had a humongous, wooden, circular board bolted above my office entrance and custom painted on it was my new logo and phone number; that's right – the obnoxious, white, winking tooth with the words Mayputz Dental - block printed on it - could now be read from a mile away! Of course, the head of the zoning board immediately phoned me to express his displeasure at my ostentatious decoration. I said two choice words to him and threatened to make the sign even larger if he persisted in his persnickety persecution of me. He never called back. Well, now I had a logo, some branded trinkets, and a sign whereby new patients could easily find me. What else? How about tackling the office demeanor and thoughtfully engaging patients for a change? And what about proper scheduling for productivity, scripted and rehearsed responses to patient queries, paying attention to the proper attire and grooming of assistants and hygienists, gratuitously asking for referrals, etc.? Those were just some of the other innovative ideas floated by the "successful" dentists out there. I was hooked and kept on reading and digesting those informative dental journals articles. More and more dental management groups like the Surly Seminars and the Prideless Institute popped up from the pages during my perusals of the magazines. They were hawking ever more elaborate marketing and monitoring services to "clueless" dentists like me. But I was learning fast on my own and devoured their spiels with a grain of salt. Some of the written advice was excellent and made sense; some was a bit nebulous, but you had to take the good with the bad. In addition, the big marketing companies promised more than run-of-the-mill continuing education and could get involved to various advanced degrees in a typical office. For a hefty fee they could "take over" a floundering practice and "manage" it, soup to nuts, complete with a third-party payroll service and utilizing their own accountants. Kind of like a franchise-sort of thing. However, the dentist would ultimately be responsible for any future failure. I didn't buy into that kind of extreme takeover but agreed to send my entire staff to at least one popular, upcoming conference to get on board this marketing locomotive. I had to do it. I felt that the dental insurance gravy train was going to end or at least not keep up with inflation. What I needed was a firm foundation of RELIABLE and LOYAL, fee-for-service patients who valued my practice, staff and me. Not just the fly-by-night insurance-card flashers. I already had plenty of them. Well, my staff came back brimming with ideas from the paid-for, weekend extravaganza, which was held on two consecutive days at a local hotel venue. They were re-energized and full of even more plans than I had previously thought of. First up was cold-mailing thousands of Welcome Wagon Neighborhood postcards to would-be patients from bought mailing lists of new homeowners in the area. And then we custom-made a phone book yellow pages advertisement and printed blue/yellow professional cards. In addition, we now offered slick office brochures with gorgeous photos of satisfied patients gracing the inside pages, complete with a thoughtfully written mission statement. And don't forget the refrigerator magnets and calendars with my name on them. Next was calling ALL our patients prior to their upcoming appointments, doing outreach programs in local malls and for kindergarten classrooms, etc. In other words, it was imperative to keep my name out there as the go-to place for dentistry! The contrived tweaks we made were all shrewd business moves and cost me a pretty penny, but I had to spend in order to get rewarded. However, now it came time to address the monies owed us. I designated a staff member (I called her the office wizard) to work in a spare "cubbyhole" solely for the purpose of gettin' the greenbacks. She was sequestered in that room all day, without being bothered, and concentrated on everything from diligent insurance coding, follow-ups on preauthorization of dental benefits, to pre-emptively phoning patients about the co-pays owed at time of checkout, etc. She and her dinky dwelling became the nerve center of the practice for eight hours a day. It was the first time someone kept track of what the hell was really going on in the office from a business, personnel and patient perspective. I hired a young lawyer to be my collections agent and he doggedly chased down deadbeats that had dodged me for years. The unexpected windfall of his perseverance coupled with the fortitude and relentless efforts of my "office wizard" were remarkable. The "extra" tidings were greatly appreciated and more than made up for any monies spent on my nascent marketing schemes.

And the old money kept coming in along with the new, and new patients kept coming in along with the old. And people actually started talking civilly to each other. Good Golly! And patients slowly began to see the professionally firm but fair machinations of receiving top notch dental care at a fair price that needed to be paid for, period. Sure, we lost a lot of nay-saying and deadbeat slackers along the way; however, my staff stayed intact, and the practice started to prosper. And not because of a congested, unreal schedule (well, that's debatable) or an unending line of dental insurance bullshitters but because of a buttload of savvy and sophisticated protocols I had put in place to garner respect and payment. Not all of the "revolutionary" ideas worked out and it was always an evolutionary process, but I had managed to attract a large cross-section of differing types of patients, some with dental insurance, and some without. Nonetheless, it was all good. I never really kept track of which types of marketing worked best although I probably should have. It was a shotgun approach on my part and perhaps I was wrong and wasteful in some of my wild-eyed attempts. Did my thirty second radio ads influence anybody? Did my two-year-running and highly rated weekly, comedic, half-hour, local public television show about health-related topics, which featured hometown celebrities, generate potential clients? I don't know. But I do know that after my total immersion into all facets of marketing, I provoked tremendous amounts of resentment from fellow highbrow dentists who saw my attempts as nothing more than giving away cheap *tchotchkes* and romping in campy theater, akin to the old Crazy Eddie commercials of yesteryear. Only I wasn't the one insane! Nevertheless, I knew I had turned the financial corner once and for all when my yellow tee shirts and black shot glasses, both emblazoned with the slogan "I Survived Dr. Mayputz," were featured in a local newspaper article about the latest marketing gimmicks used by successful dentists. It was all in good fun and patients loved to be in on the gags. And it gave me yet another buzz in the community, much to the chagrin, disdain and envy of the staid, general dentists around me. Did I go over the top by the late nineties? Perhaps, but it was all based on necessary survival and not vanity. Honest! Do I still do that now? No, I am a part-time employee prosthodontist with no stake in my current workplace. And there is no need to actively solicit new patients while coercing the existing ones to pay. The dental practice is a prosperous, well-oiled machine that has been efficiently running on all cylinders for decades and I am grateful and happy to be a part of it. I was thinking about that fact the other night as I poured myself a shot of Old Grand Dad bourbon into a leftover shot glass from 1993. I survived myself – good times!

15

Bite Me

Bud S. was referred to me by a slew of his General Electric buddies who, as a group of goofy blue-collar men, took a dental shine to me en masse. I appreciated their humorous natures, raunchy hunting and fishing escapades, and willingness to trust me with their oral needs. It was a winning combination for all concerned. And then there was Bud S., the outlier, the melancholy and egotistical bad apple of the bunch. During his introductory and cursory visit, he bemoaned the fact that he was only willing to become my patient because his co-workers were tired of him bellyaching about his teeth. He had not seen a dentist in many years and appeared highly apprehensive and volatile. He was the kind of guy whose buttons did not have to be pushed very far to get a violent response from, both verbally and physically. However, he had agreed to become my patient and I grudgingly obliged, basically as a favor to his cohort of pals. Ordinarily I would have instantly dismissed him from my practice and made up some bogus excuse for not being able to properly treat him but there I was, a *schmuck* about to treat a *schmuck*! He opened his pie-hole and I was not surprised at what I saw:

a severely collapsed bite from a lifetime of tooth grinding, no doubt at least partially related to his caustic personality. Also, the lower front bridge was all metal, devoid of any porcelain that had previously covered it. It was also tilted inwards from years of misaligned occlusal stresses. My initial observation also revealed a dentition that was largely deformed and damaged. Nevertheless, he lamented that the metallic-looking lower bridge bothered him the most and adroitly asked me if I could fix it. "Could I?" I wondered to myself. This was a prosthodontic clusterfuck and he was a screwball, but I was a prosthodontist dammit; I had to do something. I couldn't just bail and fail. After a detailed examination, x-ray evaluation and detailed work-up, I carefully outlined and noted the best treatment options for Bud. S. and awaited his answer at a subsequent appointment. Our office had also sent in an estimate of benefits for a lower anterior six-unit bridge to his dental insurance company. In addition, I had the staff allow me enough time in case we proceeded with some type of initial restorative procedures. The day arrived and I laid it on the line for him. However, while professionally explaining the need for advanced comprehensive dentistry to correct his occlusal discrepancy (his bite needed to be raised) with a multitude of crowns and bridgework, he burst out laughing. It was most inappropriate to stop my spiel with sarcastic guffaws. He really was a pompous a-hole and very disrespectful. I was pissed off and glowered at him. "No offense Doc., but all I can afford is to replace my bottom bridge with a new one. That's it. No bite raises, no extensive digging around. Got it?" he growled. Oh, I got it alright and felt like punching him. This jackass was starting to get deep under my skin and I did not like it. On top of that, I could not grant his wish with dental certainty. Fabricating a new lower bridge without first opening his bite was next to impossible, and to increase his bite he needed prosthetic work on all his other teeth in order to maintain it. Dental occlusion is an all-inclusive phenomenon. You can't raise up one tooth without it affecting all the others. That's how the teeth work. I just didn't have the proper space available to remake his existing bridge into a functional and ESTHETIC fixed prosthesis. And that's when his corrosive character went to work on me. "You call yourself a specialist?" he jeered. "Ha, you just don't want to do it 'cause you're afraid. Plus, my insurance company approved it, so there," he sardonically chuckled. "God-fucking-dammit," I silently thought to myself. He was right, though; a new bridge was indeed authorized. At that point I definitely should have politely but firmly dismissed him, however, I did not. My bloated dental ego would not let me off the hook and somehow that pissy patient knew it as well. On top of that the dental insurance consultant had given it the green light, so....I rethought my options and believed that if I could shave a little off the insides of his top front incisors, I might have enough wiggle room to make a lower bridge without having to cap the remainder of his teeth. I prayed to any god out there and hoped that stealing from Peter to pay Paul would work out. And so, we proceeded with that modified plan. It wasn't ideal but it would quickly grant his desire and I could quickly get him out of my hair, when I used to have some. However, his bite collapse was so severe that I ended up cutting off more enamel than I would have liked from his natural upper teeth and started to sweat. If I overcut them and exposed the nerves, then they would need root canals and crowns. I did not believe Bud S. would easily comprehend the added necessary therapy or forgive me for foisting unexpected and expensive dentistry on him. It was all so demoralizing and needlessly stressful. I was already way behind schedule and my dental assistant P. and staff had gone to lunch as I alone kept gingerly grinding away on Bud S. I eventually and successfully removed his lower faulty bridge and managed to not overly maim his upper choppers as I laid down my dental drill in exhaustion and exultation. And then I exhaled! Now for the easy parts: impressions, cementing

89

the temporary bridge, and then patient dismissal. I was really looking forward to the latter. Two weeks later the completed bridge was inserted uneventfully, and no undue sensitivity materialized from the altered upper teeth. Nevertheless, the patient hated it. Shocker! "It's so tiny, I can hardly see it and it is pinching my gums," he loudly grumbled. In all fairness, it WAS rather small. Although well-made and accurately seated under extremely trying oral circumstances, the patient did not see things that way and threatened not to pay his dental insurance co-pay. Shocker! At that point I did not care as he left the office still spouting out hateful and derogatory words from his newly restored mouth. And true to form he never returned or settled his monetary balance with me. Whether it was a cunning and premeditated plan of his from the beginning I do not know. All I know is that his insurance payment portion barely covered my dental laboratory expense and I basically broke even on the case. I had broken my back to satisfy that bum and got jerked around instead. And I never went after him for what he owed me. What was the point? Even if I had sent his account to collections, I would not have collected any deserving banknotes. He undoubtedly would have fought it and possibly made trouble for me. It was better to swallow my pride and walk away from that painful dental debacle than dig my heels in and fight. To add insult to injury, his jovial comrades gradually stopped coming to my office on a regular basis and then disappeared altogether a short time later. Dentally, I had done nothing wrong to any of them; sometimes life is not fair. But I'm sure that Bud S.'s continued bad-mouthing of me had soured the goodwill that I had painstakingly mustered among his fellow workers and that alone may have made them leave my practice. All it takes is one rotten apple.

16

Pre-Holiday Crush

I wished it was just an annual aberration before each major U.S. holiday, however, it was not. As sure as rain, and like precision clockwork, the days preceding Thanksgiving, Christmas, Purim, Rosh Hashanah, Yom Kippur, Hannukkah, etc., saw all my varied offices over the years filled with "emergency patients." Whether I was the owner or an employee-dentist at the time made no difference. And unlike the anticipated crowds because of a hallowed American event such as Black Friday, Caucasian-challenged Friday for the politically correct, the unscheduled stampede of patients that beat a path to my office for days prior to federally sanctioned time off was overwhelming. If there was a blockbuster national vacation coming up, certain peeps came out of the woodwork not only to get last minute dental work done but to try my patience as well. First, a side note: Dr. B., a *menschy* dentist for whom I worked part-time during dental school would always respond with this exclamation should someone ask how he was doing: "Could be busier." It was a punchy throwaway line that implied humility and his status as a no-nonsense, nose-to-the-grindstone practitioner. It also prevented further questioning by patients. But in reality, he was insanely busy, successful, and a proud dentist. However, he never wanted to jinx himself and purposely lowballed his achievements to "stay hungry." Dr. B. never wanted to grow complacent or arrogant for fear of a downturn in his practice. I remembered his catchphrase and embodied it during my early dental years. It was good to have tremendous patient traffic and to be making lots of legal tender. Nevertheless, I tempered any leaking hubris by realizing that all my outward dental attainments could vanish with one major lawsuit, a bout of bad health, etc. So I stayed humbly hungry and was eager to treat vast swaths of patients on a daily basis. But around the holidays, things got more than a little overheated, even for me. Let me explain: My Tuesday was jam packed, the hygienists' schedules were overflowing, and the phone kept ringing off the hook. Memorial Day was fast approaching, and the front office staff tried in vain to squeeze in as many "toothaches" as possible during the intervening days leading up to it. Now, I know all about emergencies; they happen to us all. My family and I have had them occur to us at inopportune times. We have all suffered from accidents that warranted medical and dental intervention afterhours, on weekends and, yes, just before or during a vacation. But when do dental emergency visits become abusive or obnoxious? Is the patient who waited for months with an obvious abscess, only to beg to be seen before his planned trip to Disneyland, a knucklehead for waiting so long? Is the patient who broke his premolar weeks ago now a candidate for an extensive restorative procedure within a ten-minute allotted time slot? I surveyed my Tuesday patient load and shook my head in disgust. I knew what was coming and could predict the onslaught to follow. Some of the added people truly had unfortunate and untimely dental shit happen to them, the others were just abusing my staff and me because of their shitty, egocentric personalities. How else can I say it? And some of the worst offenders were not even patients of mine, but "off the street" urchins looking for a quick fix and an even quicker getaway. And it was a false narrative to assume that all those "rescued" people would be so appreciative as to become patients of record and long-term, loyal clients in my practice. I would be bending over backwards for little gain, both financially and dentally. Many Shylocks would also flash an insurance card in my face in hopes of not paying a dime for services rendered. In all the commotion of days like that, I'm sure multiple enterprising patients received free dentistry, albeit in a minimalist fashion. I did not have the time to repair a giant dental mess and usually did the best I could to alleviate pain and suffering, and to cobble together broken parts and pieces so people could masticate again. My regular patients lost out on those out-of-control days because I was pulled in so many directions and into three operatories at once. So besides losing my temper all day while the telephones were buzzing, I kept thinking that there must be a better way. And there was, at least for me. After one more July Fourth debacle, I cavalierly decided not to schedule anyone for a week prior to any holiday. All days and time windows would be wide open. Anyone could come in as needed, at any time. My staff grew concerned that we would lose much money because of my seemingly temperamental and knee-jerk reaction to being so stupidly overtaxed on those certain days. It was a valid point because our country does celebrate a good number of times. I would go broke if all we did was wait around and treat lost fillings, fractured teeth and give out antibiotic and pain-relieving prescriptions. So, I compromised. We would appoint a lower number of patients for both the hygienists and me for every pre-holiday week, take our time to unhurriedly treat each person properly, see the emergency visitors as needed, and still make a profit. And I made it happen. Everyone was happy except for that fifty-ish redneck Mr. Gruffie. He plunked down in my chair the day before New Year's one year and exclaimed, "I cracked my tooth, Doc. Can you pull the sucker out right now?" "You know, crack kills," I jokingly responded. He didn't think that was funny and thought even less of me when I asked if he cracked it on hard water. "No, I was eating plain vanilla yogurt last month and heard a crunch," he mumbled. "Oh, another liar. And it happened last month, and you had all this time to come in but did not, you idiot," I thought to myself. And since when do rednecks eat yogurt, anyway? It's more likely that he was drunkenly opening a Bud beer bottle with his teeth again when the tooth snapped. An ensuing radiograph and dental examination confirmed a damning diagnosis. He had a *schmutz-mouth* and actually needed more than just this one tooth extracted. He wasn't a regular customer and only came in when in discomfort. I told him the best I could do was give him an antibiotic prescription to quell the infection and to take Motrin for the pain. He needed to be referred to an oral surgeon for the difficult molar extraction. Mr. Gruffie was outraged, as I expected he would be. And instead of feeling embarrassment or being apologetic for his poor and neglected oral condition, this surly fellow was giving me some guff. I promptly stood up and showcased my athletically chiseled physique and large biceps before stating coldly, "You need to see an oral surgeon, Mr. Gruffie. There is nothing else I can do for you today." I was prepared to physically fight that bastard, Honest Injun! My dental assistant thought for sure there would be fisticuffs involved and backed away into a neutral corner just in case of trouble. But nothing deleterious occurred. Perhaps my daily gym-work and tennis playing had paid off. Mr. Gruffie eyeballed me towering over him with clenched fists and backed off on the angry meter. He grumpily took the two prescriptions and stalked out of the office, without letting the staff make a referral appointment to a local oral surgeon for him. Of course I had the time for an extraction, but it would have been difficult for me. And suppose I could not have done it and abdicated halfway through the procedure. Then what: A belligerent patient in great discomfort to be sent to a closed oral surgeon's office on New Year's Eve to bail me out? Ha, ha. I did the right thing with my treatment plan. Unfortunately, Mr. Gruffie did not play ball although perhaps he did find a sucker dentist to yank his lower right first molar just before the ball dropped in Times Square? Maybe. But the larger story here is that dentists are dentally assaulted daily by the likes of "entitled" Mr. Gruffie, regardless of the involvement of holidays or not. I realize that pain is pain but come on man; most dentists cannot treat a lifetime of dental neglect, or perform a very difficult procedure, during a limited time slot just because the patient wishes it so. Common decency, mutual respect and logic should dictate treatment but often do not. What else can I say?

17

Crazy is as Crazy Does

I don't know if someone tattled on me or not. Either way, the three, somber, city-building inspectors showed up one fine morning and shook their collective heads while inspecting my practice premises. They told me nothing as they vacated, still shaking their noggins in unison. That unannounced visit, combined with the extreme pressure I felt from the building's out-of-state owner to quickly buy said structure, caused me to re-evaluate my priorities, location and lease. I had inked a long-term deal with him to eventually purchase the property and was paying a pretty penny for the privilege of being a tenant. I was paying off the bank and the note held by the previous dentist/practice owner, as well. In other words, I was strapped to the gills in debt and here was the building owner constantly badgering me to buy his huge monstrosity. But I kept stalling him because there was no way I was ready. The Florida-based landlord, though a fellow Estonian by ancestry, was a pistol-packing SOB oral surgeon who was basically run out of town years ago for performing shoddy and unethical dentistry. And he reputedly carried a gun in case his jilted ex-wife confronted him whenever he visited the area. At least that's what he told me on numerous occasions when he surreptitiously appeared at my office. What was wrong with him? Oh, well. With all that hanging over my head, I decided to "technically" sell my practice and quietly abdicated my mini fiefdom on upper Union Street. I went due north, to a burgeoning suburban community called Milfton Park, which was rapidly filling up with White Flight, an upper crusty populace of serious male breadwinners and their predominantly stay-at-home wives. The mostly White newbie suburbanites came from the surrounding crime-ridden and blackened communities of Skankectady, Troilet and the State Capitol, Smallbany. The public schools in this onetime wilderness were topnotch as were the beautiful developments springing up all over former cow pastures. I had secured a vacant former dental office on a main drag, signed the lease, mailed the old keys to that pushy landlord in Wacahoota, Florida, and dragged my kit and caboodle out of Skankectady. The new rent was much cheaper allowing me the luxury to purchase brand new dental equipment. Score! But then the shit hit the fan. I had effectively broken the old contract and my former landlord was less than pleased. He threatened retaliation and to "shoot me up," as he unpleasantly shouted into the blower. I calmly held the rotary phone receiver to my ear and, in my best Mae West impression, sarcastically said that "he could come up and see me some time," if he wanted ME to bust a cap in HIS ass. I also owned firearms and he knew it. However, I never carried a rod on me nor was I lying awake at night waiting for him, unlike his supposedly "crazed" ex-wife. He never showed up, at least not that I knew of, and I never heard from that scoundrel again. A few weeks later a reliable source related to me that a "for sale" sign had been placed on the berm in front of the building I had left. And then the same person laughingly told me that he later witnessed a caravan of hazmat-suit-covered men descend on that very same compound and raze it to the ground. The former evangelical church, which was long ago converted into a giant dental office, was now a smoldering heap of ash. God sure does work in mysterious ways. Or maybe the Antichrist was involved? And that asshole landlord had desperately wanted me to purchase it? Did he know it was distressed and about to be demolished? Maybe so. What a piece of scum he was. I had dodged a ruinous financial bullet and possibly a real one from his .22 caliber peashooter as well. Nevertheless, the needless agitation that he and my subsequent move caused me had been intense. Fortunately, I did not start imbibing recklessly or start abusing drugs, and I would have been justified if I had. Anyhow, I was settling into my new digs as former patients realized that I had moved and they slowly began the five-mile northerly hike to rejoin me and my practice. But I also had a ton of new faces showing up. Unknowingly, I had picked a great location and time period to set up shop and felt that the dental gods might finally be smiling down on me. But you know what they say, "Wherever you go, there you are." Did I somehow attract all the losers and lunatics? Was there a sign on the office door and on my forehead that read "All loonies please enter here?" Some days it felt like that. Anyway, Mrs. Diamante W. was a new transplant to Milfton Park; she was a homemaker and of Greek descent. She was actually born in Greece, married a U.S. service member who was stationed there, and then became a citizen of our country. She had a bit of an accent going on but so what? She had a few mildly carious teeth that needed attention and a poorly fitting partial upper denture that warranted replacement; nothing unusual and well within my wheelhouse of ability. I casually outlined the proposed dental treatment and we agreed upon a financial plan and a realistic timetable to complete her oral needs. And then insanity popped up out of nowhere. At the very next visit, as I was preparing to locally anesthetize the damaged teeth and do a whole bunch of fillings in one sitting, Diamante started to act in an unorthodox fashion. Did it have something to do with her Greek Orthodox faith? Perhaps it was the anxiety of the moment, but, regardless, it scared the bejesus out of me. Let's put it this way: alternating between professing her love for me out loud and then shouting for help and then caterwauling at the top of her lungs in Greek consonants was abnormal, am I right? But instead of a panic reaction, maybe she was having a stroke or other medical emergency? I couldn't be sure as I repeatedly scanned her medical history and tried to interpret the interspersed Hellenic ramblings and body gesticulations. She was bobbing to and fro in the chair and I was petrified. On my command my assistant P. raced to the waiting room to fetch her husband and reportedly saw frozen and frightened faces on the patients there. Obviously, they were hearing the same thing I was, regardless of the easy listening elevator music blaring at them from the speakers in the ceiling. Luckily her husband bolted upright and sprinted back to my operatory, closely following my trembling assistant. I saw a huge Black dude approach Diamante and for a split second did not link them as a couple. You see, I had never met him before. Did conservative Greek women marry Black men? Did her father know of their union? All those politically incorrect and racist thoughts exited my brain as Mr. W. soothingly stroked her legs while introducing himself to me. He then curtly explained that his wife was tripolar and had purposely failed to mention that on her health history sheet because she feared I would not understand. I thought he misspoke and said, "You mean bipolar, don't you?" as my adrenaline-induced heart kept trying to leap out of my chest. As Diamante quieted down, Mr. W. explained, "On a good day, she is polar but then goes ape shit crazy and completely bypasses bipolar. That's why she is tripolar." I stared at him in disbelief. Was he making up that incredulous crapola? I had never heard of such a thing before. "You mean she TRIES hard to be polar but sometimes messes up and becomes tripolar?" I jokingly asked. Mr. W. just grimaced sadly at me. "Could she be cyclothymic? You know, suffer from mood swings during the day, unlike having true bipolar manic and depressive episodes?" I further queried him, this time with a serious expression on my face. "I don't think so, she is so fucked up that all our family and friends call her condition tripolar," Mr. W. sorrowfully insisted. "And she doesn't take any medications for this?" I dubiously asked. "No, there is no cure for being from that part of Greece," he nonchalantly replied. What? What part of Greece was she from? Was he for real? I didn't know whether to laugh, cry or hurl. This conversation had gone south in a hurry and I decided to shut up. And then a quickie daydream hit me. Perhaps if I had practiced tennis more as a child and had the required talent, maybe I could have been a professional tennis player and now would be happily retired with millions instead of sitting there as a demoralized and defeated dentist. Then I snapped out of it and surveyed the surreal scene before me and knew the rest of my day would suck as well. And I would have to apologize to the remainder of my patient patients for being tardy. I exhaled and sank down in my dentist's chair with nary a comedic thought in my blasted mind. I had my dental assistant escort the husband and wife out of the operatory and an appointment was made for another time, hopefully with her behaving better. As I stupidly sat there in a stupor, while listening to her tearfully mumble an apology as she left, I wondered if what I heard from Mr. W. was just psycho-babble to cover up for a hysterical and mentally unstable spouse or did she indeed have a genuine mental illness for which there were no medicaments or therapy? Was it a malady which only affected Greek women? "No way in hell," I said to myself. However, I had no additional answers as my dental assistant P. seated the next victim. I composed myself and started the familiar spiel of greetings, followed by Novocain, followed by numbness, followed by …., you know. And for those of you curious as to what eventually transpired, here is the rest of the story, as Paul Harvey used to say: Between outbreaks of outlandish conniption fits and blood curdling shrieking to petting my thighs in suggestive sexual foreplay, I somehow managed to "tame the beast" and accomplished the required dental work. Although struggling mightily against a mental adversary I was never taught about in dental school, I repaired Diamante's dentition with aplomb. Even the new partial upper denture fit her like a glove. I had insisted that Mr. W. be present in the room with me during each "performance" by his wife, and that compounded to the palpable anguish hanging in the surrounding atmosphere. Regardless of taking deep, cleansing breaths, many times that "heavy air" almost suffocated me. In addition, all that nervous tension left me exhausted after every visit. Dentistry is hard on a good day; it wasn't supposed to be THIS hard! I never found out what really ailed her as she and her husband refused to divulge any hidden medical truths at succeeding appointments. I finished her mouth, yet she almost finished me. Satisfied, they left happy; I was happy they left!

18

"I Don't Want a Damn X-Ray!"

"But Mrs. R.," I sarcastically rebutted, "Who am I, Superman? I don't have x-ray vision and we need to see why your tooth is aching." "No," she emphatically stated and started to get apoplectic in the dental chair. "They are expensive, unnecessary, give off way too much radiation and cause cancer," she further added. Oh, boy. I was a relative old-timer at this *game* by now and yet it seemed like only yesterday that I heard that same retort from another bellicose patient. With great restraint I tried to explain that ultra-low radiation, digital, periodic radiographs (x-rays) were necessary to properly diagnose carious decay/jaw-related problems and to avoid potential dental malpractice because of an error of omission on the dentist's part. "So, you're just covering your ass even though you might not really need it?" she screamed at me. "Can't you use the ones I had done when I had my cleaning last year? What's wrong with you dentists? Always in it for the money!" she snarled. Causing cancer and illicitly making money, is that what dentistry boiled down to? How demoralizing. Then I suddenly remembered that she was a long-timer and always behaved this way as I turned sideways to my computer screen and reread the copious previous notes about her. "Mrs. R.," I repeated in a strained voice, "I know your tooth hurts, but we have to know why and last years' full mouth series will not tell us. We need a fresh x-ray to determine what's wrong." My blood pressure and anxiety had risen right on cue because of that belligerent old biddy as she folded up her arms across her chest and then exclaimed, "Well, since I'm trapped here you might as well get it over with, and I hope it's not a root canal because I don't have that kind of money!" She was my first patient of the day, an emergency at that, and already was trying my patience. I motioned to my quaking assistant P. to take the x-ray of the offending tooth and call me when it was ready. I had won the battle of wits for now and could hopefully diagnose her dental discomfort. But what if she had insisted on no radiation whatsoever? Then what? Have her sign a medical release form, which she most likely would not have agreed to, and try to poke and prod at her sore tooth hoping to visually or manually detect a deficit? Sometimes an obvious hole in the enamel or a broken tooth can easily be seen but oftentimes there is an internal infection or trauma that only a radiograph can detect. Hypothetically speaking, let's say I did not take one, discharged her and the problem escalated. And let's say she consulted another dentist who somehow successfully irradiated her tooth and diagnosed a raging infection, etc. Who would get the blame? Yours truly, of course. During the ensuing malpractice trial she would NOT utter something like, "Yeah, it's my own fault, judge. I should have let Dr. Mayputz take the damn x-ray. He is innocent of negligence!" Yeah, right. You know she would say the exact opposite, regardless of any paperwork signed by her releasing me of liability. So, come on. Dentistry is difficult enough without people giving us a difficult time to boot. I carefully studied the resultant radiographic image on the monitor, turned to face Mrs. R. and told her that nothing seemed unusual and that her pain might be due to treatable hypersensitivity or possibly to a hairline fracture of her molar. Nothing serious but worth reporting to us should her symptoms worsen. She just peered intently at me and muttered, "I told you there was nothing wrong with my tooth. Why did you have to give me cancer?" It was challenging to flummox me because I was a parboiled and relatively tough bird at this point in my career but she managed to, at least for a moment. Was it time for a funny reply or should I just grunt and dismiss her? As I thought of what to say, so many depressive and escapist thoughts flooded my mind. Maybe being a long-distance truck driver would be great right about now - all alone, no bullshit, only I, the open road and my trusty C.B. radio…. Then I came out of my mini pity-party trance and stated, "Mrs. R., why do you always give us such a difficult time? Is it my assistant's *stank*, the office music selections, the dark color of my black pants?" That did the trick. I had made her laugh. Maybe it was the stench comment? I don't know. Regardless, Mrs. R. smiled a shit-eating grin, promised to return and didn't say another word as she left. I apologized to my assistant and complimented her on being my foil and a good sport as the butt of my jokes. She just nodded and sighed deeply. We had gotten out of yet another unpleasant jam and my dental assistant appeared grateful for that, regardless of being faux-insulted by me for the umpteenth time. My boiling blood subsided to a simmer and my mental anguish started to decline before spiking again as I saw the next patient's name on the schedule. And it was only 9 a.m. I silently chuckled to myself but refused to get apathetic thoughts. As soon as a dentist starts not to care or writes off every "crazy" patient as being truly crazy, that's when things go awry for the practice. Patients can always sense if the dentist's heart isn't in it or when she/he is not being genuine. However, empathy can cause great pain and suffering for the doctor. So what are we dentist-types to do? Hit the bottle at 9 a.m., pop some pills, take some deep breaths, psycho-analyze the situation and self-prescribe a psychic tonic for our mind, or just grin and bear it? Most of us take the sucker punches, vocalize some feeble verbiage, move on with ulcer-lined intestinal fortitude, and do not feel the need to jump out a window so early in the morning! Hopefully, Mrs. R.'s kind of recurring and insulting office nonsense does not reach a critical mass and result in self harm to the dentist. Am I being overly melodramatic? Perhaps, but I keep hearing unwarranted, unpleasant adjectives from patients even to this day; and they still psychologically sting.

19

I'm Dying

We have all heard someone utter those profound words in jest, haven't we? And most likely they came from the types of people who are known kidders. The other candidates for that kind of dark humor are ones who crave attention, are obvious hypochondriacs, are depressed, etc. But what about from people who really mean it? Probably not so often I would guess. Mrs. Dungfree had been coming to my office for a few months for regular, minor, restorative dental treatments. You know, a filling here and there but no big work. Each time that I even mildly suggested that she should invest some time and money into more substantial oral therapy to improve her chewing ability she would utter the same thing: "I'm dying Dr. Mayputz. Just patch me up as best you can to keep me going for now." And more expensive dentistry did not happen in her mouth! I recall scouring her medical history and questioning her about any recent diagnoses that I did not know about. Everything seemed in order and appeared fairly mundane except for an anti-hypertensive medication she was taking. Did she have cancer and was embarrassed to tell me? Was her heart frail and about to fail? Was she an intuitive Reiki Master and destined for death in the very near future? I did not get any easy rejoinders as I did not ask her those kinds of probing questions. Perhaps I should have. She was all of sixty-five, always well-dressed for appointments and seemed spritely for her age. However, although a widow, I would not say she was merry. Anyhow, her dental gamesmanship continued for a time; I strongly suspected that it was all an act, kind of like the recurring "fatal heart attack" comedy bit on *Sanford and Son*. Comedian Redd Foxx played iconic curmudgeon Fred G. Sanford on that hit TV show. He would routinely clutch at his chest in fake agony while saying he was "having The Big One" and threatened to die so he could join his beloved Elizabeth in heaven. Was Mrs. Dungfree a female Fred Sanford? It seemed so, as I would jokingly tell my staff after each of her visits. Anyhow, one day my dental assistant just happened to mention that we had not seen her in a while. So, I had my receptionist call her at home. Oh, we got an answer all right. Mrs. Dungfree's daughter had picked up the phone and stated that her mother had died a few weeks prior, just as she had predicted she would. Even her own daughter knew she was going to pass away. It just couldn't be or could it? I could not believe the news and it caused me great anxiety and distress. All that time that I was joshing Mrs. Dungfree about kicking off and yet she was sincere all along and finally did it. And it wasn't suicide. I was such a *maroon* and mortified at my flippant and unempathetic approach to her. But what did she really die of? Alas, I never found out. My curiosity did not go any farther because it was not my professional duty to pry deeper. I probably could have thoroughly questioned her daughter or even asked her doctor but then I would have been in violation of HIPAA patient privacy laws, so I dropped any queries I might have had. And that was that. But the next time someone "healthy" tells me that she/he is dying, I will believe it!

20

Bad News

How many times have I had to tell a patient that a tooth could not be saved, had a large hole in it, needed a root canal or many large bills were required to get the entire mouth back in shape? Thousands of times, I reckon. And it is never a pleasant task or one you get used to, no matter how many times you have done it. I find myself the bearer of bad news multiple times a day, often relating negative findings to already nervous and disbelieving patients. Even a perplexing diagnosis of "I don't know" can be dentally devastating to a hurting patient. Mr. Burppoe had been sent to me by his conscientious wife, who was a longtime patient in my practice. He sat down rather anxiously in the dreaded hot seat not knowing what to expect. It was his first visit with me, and I figured I'd take some bitewing x-rays, do an oral exam, plot the course of treatment, and schedule him for future appointments as needed. He cautiously tilted his head back and bellowed, "My wife sent me. Nothing hurts, but I think I have a few small holes in my teeth. Oh, and nothing personal Doc., but I hate all dentists!" Now, what do you suppose a normal reaction should be to a comment like that? Should all dentists be trained psychotherapists and verbally diffuse a potentially deleterious situation, or should all dentists have a trained sense of humor and laugh it off, or should dentists be skilled in fighting techniques and be allowed to physically assault the patient because he/she is such an asshole? Unfortunately, I was not specifically mentored in any of those methods. Instead, I gritted my teeth and carefully examined his choppers while peering at his x-rays on the monitor behind him and, was aghast at the damage done to his dentition. His mouth was a dump, not to mention the reeking alcohol stench on his breath, yellow tobacco stains on his back molars and piled up tartar on the insides of his front incisors. It was revolting to witness and by rights he should have been in intense oral pain. Now whether he weathered earlier swellings and discomfort, I do not know. But he should have been in intractable discomfort based on all the humongous craters in his molars alone. I was flabbergasted and tried to be as diplomatic as possible while telling him the bad news. However, first he interjected and slurred, "Hope it's not too bad, Doc., now don't hurt me!" His obvious psychologically distrusting nature radiated to me and I started to perspire. He didn't want to be there, and it showed. I didn't want to be there at that point either! Here was a good-ole-country boy whose fastidious wife wanted completely dentally overhauled, and yet he acted as if a few fillings would suffice. Now, this wasn't my first rodeo and I decided to dive right in with my examination results. After a few minutes of patiently explaining all the time, effort and funds that were necessary to get him shipshape, he suddenly glared at me and exclaimed, "Are you fuckin' kidding me? Are all you guys in it for the money? I told you nothing hurts. Weren't you listening?" A younger version of me would have cowered and started stammering and stuttering while trying to educate this Neanderthal about his oral maladies. That's what they taught us idiots to do in dental school. But I also knew from piss-poor past experiences that long-winded dental explanations were rarely commensurate to the patient's eventual level of understanding and acceptance. And after putting up with thousands of such lousy louts, I found myself losing patience with patients like him. It just wasn't worth my sanity to argue with a coon chasing, bass fishing, roughneck who thought he was being chiseled (literally and figuratively). I abruptly left the operatory to cool off but not before telling my assistant to go over his findings one more time. Perhaps a feminine approach was needed with this character? And you know, it worked. When I returned after a few minutes, he had become a different man. Conciliatory and polite, he seemed to be coming out of his drunken stupor and apologized for being so rude. I was quick to tell him that there was no guarantee that any dentistry performed on him would initially be pain free. He was puzzled at my proclamation and seemed to be ruminating on the business axiom of "you broke it, you fix it." I hurriedly interjected that his very deep carious cavities would not be amenable to quickie fillings and would most likely need additional dentistry such as root canals or extractions. Nevertheless, he acquiesced to a watered-down version of the dentistry needed and we slowly began. After multiple visits of writhing (on my part) and painstaking (on his part) dental treatment we arrived at a mutual ending and it had not cost him a fortune as he had once feared. Of course, he was now missing many formerly non-restorable teeth. But at least the remaining ones had been periodontally treated, polished up and were restored strongly enough to crimp lead sinkers with whenever he decided to go fishin' again. Mr. Burppoe was happy, his wife was happy, and I was just happy that things had not escalated into verbal or physical hostilities at the outset of our time together. It could have been nasty; oftentimes those kinds of patient encounters dented and drained me. After he left, I asked my assistant what she had said to him at the very beginning to quell his nerves and bullying persona. "Doc, I told him that if he didn't do what you said, I would call his wife and tell on him," she replied, rather smugly. I just nodded a half-hearted thank you to her and walked away.

Take a Break!

21

Staying Ahead of the Curve?

As is true of most business enterprises, you don't want to be the first or last on the block to offer a blockbuster product or service. And that sentence aptly applies to dentistry as well. However, contrary to that line of thinking why NOT stick your dental neck out and always be the first, and then brag about it through social media and advertisements? What's wrong with bringing in beaucoup bucks and new blood into your practice because you now have a whatchamacallit? Well, let's discuss this. Now, I have nothing against computers; I really don't. Today they have become our second brains and even sexual partners, but that was not the case in the nineties when their installation and usage became somewhat mandatory in dental offices. Oh, dentists knew they were coming, and they eventually did – big, boxy and barely functional. However, all the dental magazine "gurus" encouraged us "wet-fingered dentists in the trenches" not to fall behind, to get with the program and become fully paperless at once. Really? The offerings to patients would be astronomical, the business spreadsheets generated would be outstandingly accurate, and the overall space-age benefits would be immeasurable.

Really? Such was the hype, but did it jive with reality? Not really, at least not at the beginning. I desperately wished to stay ahead of the curve and invested money I did not have into a computer package consisting of two front desk monitors, keyboards, printers and CPUs (central processing units), to become the de facto free labor in the office. The name of the Chinese-made, knock-off software was SoEasyDentalYourMotherCanDoIt, or something like that. My new system would be super-duper, and patients would be duly impressed. We were now an officially computerized practice and all set to throw out the appointment book, rake in the accolades and *make bank*. What a moronic *putz* I was! The dental journal writers had made it seem logical and easy. Ha. What they conveniently neglected to mention was the steep learning curve involved, and the long nights that needed to be spent by the doctor working out all the many bugs. Dentists had to burn the proverbial midnight oil in order to get things going in the right direction during the daylight working hours. But I had no interest in another "hobby." The software manual should have been enough to peruse and comprehend but it was complicated and did not seem to apply to real life dental situations. What Chinese engineers wrote that crap; shit that no one could understand? And I even read the English version! In addition, I was not a tinkerer at heart and did not want to invest all that time into something that should be helping me and not the other way around. I longed to be like Captain Kirk and bark out futuristic orders such as, "Computer, do this and that…." and be rewarded with a warm, sultry female voice which instantly fulfilled my desires, without me mucking about with keyboard strokes or dealing with a blank screen. I was doomed and felt duped. Remember, my mindset was that of Fred Flintstone and not George Jetson when it came to new-fangled technology. But wait, perhaps if I further invested into having the software trainers come to my office, I would be all right? Nay, it was yet another capital idea that failed miserably. The company coaches came daily for a five-week period and, instead of educating my staff into becoming computer mavens, reduced them to quivering and unsure data entry clerks unable to make decisions. And the hand-written appointment book was still there, as a daily reminder of my colossal debacle! Anyway, that's how computerizing my office went at the time; in spurts and lurches with much money wasted for nothing. I never got the return on investment that I had eagerly anticipated and felt very disappointed. Fast forward thirty years and things have sure changed. Of course, now most dental offices employ a salaried "computer guy" who comes around periodically to troubleshoot, defragment discs, repair files, and gussy up the server and overall system to keep things running smoothly. And he is usually on call 24/7 for the frequent emergency crashes that occur, no matter what the software is. How naïve I had been, that with just a bit of elbow grease and boning up, I could have a modern office overnight. The joke had been on me all along. Anyway, moving right along….up and coming dental products and techniques have also been a sore subject with me. When do you purchase that gizmo, gadget or new cement? Or should you buy it at all? And will it truly help your patients, regardless of the imaginary demand out there? And what if a smart-alecky patient comes in asking for something you don't currently offer? Holy hell, you had better get on the ball and start buying lest you fall further behind and become known as an antiquated office. No pressure or stress there! Old Dr. J., a long-retired dentist, became my steady patient in the nineties and always had a few choice dental stories to share. One of his favorites was to mention his large closet full of "new and improved" dental objects that he had accumulated over the years. He used most of them once and then they just gathered dust. They were each originally supposed to revolutionize dentistry and he fell for the hype at the time, much like all of us do. But alas, only a handful became mainstays of dental practice and the rest of the useless artifacts were relegated to the obscure dustbin of dental history. Dr. J. estimated that he had spent well over thirty thousand dollars in total (that was a lot of money in the fifties and sixties) to stay up-to-date and ahead of the curve. He often jokingly asked me if I wanted to purchase his closet full of useless clutter, and then we would have a good laugh together when I sarcastically answered yes. And not only did many "dental Segways" not pan out, but oftentimes much ballyhooed techniques and actual dental prostheses did no better. The "new," inexpensive Maryland Bridge of the late '8os could be glued onto teeth thereby closing an unsightly space. "No more drilling, no more cutting down enamel, no more pain for the patient!" Holy shit! What an endorsement and what a cheap technique with a positive outcome. How could you go wrong? Ha! Of course dentists, including me, started fabricating them like mad; most failed within five years time, however. The glue simply did not hold, and angry patients wanted their greenbacks back. Was that the evidence-based dentistry that we were supposed to uphold as practitioners of the oral arts? Ha! Burned and hornswoggled again! But wait a second. What about those gorgeous, glass/ceramic crowns that were hawked and talked about in women's magazines and in our dental journals during that same time period? The "new" Dicor crowns would be super fantastic! No more opacity, no more metal showing through at the crown margins and no more patients bellyaching about the artificial aesthetics of their front caps. Yay, finally a winning combination of increased wealth for dentists and a guaranteed cosmetic solution for picky people. Not so fast *homey*. Most failed within a few years. Hoodwinked again! The material did not hold up and fractured at an alarming rate. Plus the dental cements used at the time, which slightly internally expanded, also contributed to the crowns' untimely demise. After getting bushwhacked by those newfangled Maryland bridges and Dicor crowns, I backed off at accumulating the "must have" whatsits and widgets for my office, no matter what the dental *schmucks* down the street allegedly advertised that they possessed. Dental microscopes, in-office bleaching lights, painless lasers that can replace dental drills (yeah, right), in-office, one-hour, 3-D, crown-making milling machines, etc. are some of the "latest and greatest" thingamabobs in the dental world. Can you still practice fine dentistry without them? I think so. Will they stick around for a while and become long-haulers like some unfortunate Wuhan Flu patients, or will they be found at future flea markets? Who knows? My final thoughts are these: Some toothy techniques and prosthodontic prostheses are okay, but some will get you nowhere. It's just hard to tell the difference at the time. And buyers beware: don't end up with a trunk full of junk either! Amen, and Awoman. Just TRYING to be inclusive and politically correct; you know how I am.

22

Confessions

Hey, I'm not a Catholic priest. I don't want to hear about your private, guilt-ridden troubles and turmoil. I'm only a lowly dentist, with my latex-gloved fingers in your mouth. Please stop talking so I can finish! Too late, the vocalizations had commenced. Was it the atmosphere that made some patients confess and reveal their innermost thoughts? Was it me? Did I resemble a religious deity or a man of the cloth? My priestly collar was a blue surgical face mask, and my "religious garb" was a blue lab coat! Too late, they had my ear, and I wasn't deaf. Rats, I had to listen. Mrs. T. was a South Korean war bride and a real *trip*. At EVERY freakin' visit she would unload her marital woes on me. After taking off her shoes and mounting the dental chair, she would say in slightly broken English: "My no good hubband, he have women all over world. He no good!" Why did she have to tell me? She's the one who married him. Well, I treated her two teenage kids and her for years wondering what kind of a two-timing Casanova Mr. Donald T. was. Was he really a swinging chick-magnet that women swooned over? But why was I thinking those thoughts in the first place? Why was I even part of her long-running, dysfunctional soap opera life? I was just the dentist, remember? Then I finally met her husband as a new patient to the practice. After having his teeth cleaned by one of my hygienists, who was in the know, I sauntered into the room to do the exam and expected to find a virile, dashing, 007-type of man's man. I looked down and there sat a jug-eared, scrawny, pasty, pudding-faced White dude with a slight stammer. This was the Donald who had a voracious sexual appetite and who ladies found irresistible? He looked and acted more like Don Knotts than Don Juan. If he was fooling around then hats off to him, and to the women who fancied him. But I think not. My hygienist smirked the whole time during my dental examination and laughed hysterically after he left. Well, when I saw Mrs. T. again in the future, I very gently chided her that Mr. Donald T. did not strike me as being a lothario. And you know what? She took umbrage at my comments. In her mind he was a "hot" man and she had to hold onto him at all cost. Wow, I really misread that dominant marital paradigm. Fortunately, the whole family kept coming to my office for many years and Mrs. T. continued to bash her husband at every appointment as a no-good adulterer but whom she was lucky enough to have married. Sheesh! The next sleazy soliloquy is just as jarring. Big Joe was an Italian-American in his mid-thirties and always seemed to wear open V-necked shirts when in my office. And he had that solid gold ram's horn ornament attached to a thick gold chain that he proudly wore around his hairy neck. He thought himself a *player* and was always available - if the right girl was young, cute and willing (those were his words, not mine). "Hey Doc, I got back from vacation last night. Wanna hear what happened?" he said at his appointment, just as I was going to start working on a cavity in his upper right second molar. He was adequately numb but felt compelled to tell me about his recent trip before I began. So I sat back in my chair, put down the drill and listened. It turned out that he had finally gotten up the gumption to have booked a cruise ship adventure called Hedonism 1. The sales pitch was that you were guaranteed to get some *action* because everyone on board was heterosexual, young, single, and looking for the same thing, if you know what I mean. No teasing, no denial, and all the carnal chicanery that rival Carnival Cruise lines did not offer. "It was going to be great," Big Joe blurted out. But just like a typical high school dance, where hot-looking babes sashayed to the throbbing music while dorky guys were plastered alongside the wooden bleachers only imagining potential couplings, that's how this cruise went. "It was a big nothing sandwich," Big Joe mumbled. "Oh, sure there were plenty of pretty girls, but they stayed in groups for protection and it was next to impossible to peel cne off for a rumble in the hay," he dismally added. "Sc, nothing happened?" I asked. "A big fat zero," he replied as he shook his head. Time was ticking as I intimated that we had to get going to finish his treatment. But he stopped me to say, "Next year I am booking on Hedonism 2, where the girls have the option to go topless." He seemed all excited about the future trek on the open ocean while being titillated by female nipples and finally *scoring* in a consensual, carefree manner. But I'm sure there would be some catch; there always was. And knowing Big Joe, there would be outlandish and outrageous stories of alleged bait and switch, misunderstandings and skullduggery, all to thwart him in his mission to get laid. I sat there drilling away and thought of the machinations and money that Big Joe was spending once a year to get his jollies. There were plenty of "singles" bars in our area. And if he was THAT desperate, couldn't he go down to the corner of State and McClellan Streets and cheaply solicit just about any girl there that was "plying the trade?" I guess not. Perhaps the thrill of the chase, under a hot Caribbean sun, was the aphrodisiac and vibe that was missing locally. I looked forward to his return visit and to listen to more reports of anticipated sexual debauchery that never happened! The following story unfortunately involves me personally. What do you tell a middle-aged lady who keeps laying hands on you, and not in prayer or for a Reiki treatment? Good-looking Gisele was a longtime patient who had recently separated from her boyfriend and felt the need to confide in me. Please, no. Just let me fill that front tooth with the properly matched shade of composite filling and we are done. Not so fast, big boy, not so fast. "So, Doc., what's a good-looking man like you still married for?" she demurely questioned. What did that mean? Was I supposed to instantly ask her out? And then her wandering right hand started to gently stroke my right thigh in a suggestive manner. I mean, it was downright unsanitary to say the least, what with her tooth shavings all over my right pant leg and all. However, my messy trouser didn't seem to faze her and the inappropriate touching continued while she verbally revealed her need for intimacy with a "good" man. Good lord. And my horror-struck dental assistant was sitting right there! I kept moving in my chair to be out of reach of the handsy Gisele and ended up polishing her filling with my craned arms and hands over her head but with the lower part of my body nearly in the hallway. And good thing my hands don't shake because if there had been a good time for that to happen, that would have been it. And then the procedure was abruptly over. Gisele checked out the dental work in a patient mirror, stood up to formally thank me, and brusquely walked out of the operatory as if nothing had occurred. My assistant walked her to the front desk bantering small talk the whole way, with nary a mention of me or what had transpired. Maybe next time I would pretend to enthusiastically take her up on her offer? Perhaps not. There was no need to ask for trouble. I was the so-called "professional" in the room and maybe she was just having one of those days? Sometimes inhibitions break down and emotions can be expressed in various ways and at different times under dental duress. And dentistry can be an unforgiving bitch; the same probably goes for groping Gisele.

23

The Schedule

Ulrich Leonard Tölle, the formerly well-educated, unemployed, clinically depressed, bullshitter-turned-"enlightened," New Age prophet Eckhart Tölle, has written a number of best-selling books on spirituality. Self-awareness and living in the moment and deriving pleasure from both, while constantly analyzing yourself from a third person perspective, are the crux of his teachings. I know, I've read some of his books too! Tölle's distillation of established religious and spiritual axioms into readily readable teachings is comparable to how Confucius got undeserved credit by compiling esoteric historical texts and rambling parables of his time into commonsense sayings that the common Chinaman could understand. Anyhow, now that I have essentially panned both of those gurus in one sentence, it's time for the gist of this story. In one of Tölle's many volumes he states that there are three courses of action one can take when confronted with an unrelenting problem. Loosely paraphrased, they are: Acceptance, change the circumstances, or run away. My daily dental schedule was my "problem" and for years I desperately tried to make it work for and not against me!

But it was a futile battle that I bravely fought yet constantly lost, similar in context to the punished Greek God Prometheus, whose immortal liver regrew every night after being eaten in the daytime by Zeus's eagle. That was my lot: a dizzying daily avalanche of patients plus the overwhelming side-book emergencies which made me feel like I was on roller-skates, with a reprieve only coming at night. And the ensuing *daze* brought more of the same: the constant drumbeat and pressure of staying on time and trying to do no harm, while performing my dental *shtick* for the paying public. "You should be so busy," old Dr. B., from my dental school days, would have probably said with a slightly mocking Yiddish lilt to his voice. And it was true, damn true, as legendary WWE wrestler Kurt Angle would say! But while grateful for staying financially solvent and being consistently booked solid for two months, the insanely hectic, frenetic pace was getting to me bigtime. Something had to be done before I completely fried my brain or became an alcoholic. However, after scrutinizing Tölle's three pillars of resolution it became obvious that I could not run away, nor could I accept the status quo any longer. So that left changing the circumstances as the only logical solution for me. But how was I going to do it? Better dentists than I could not solve the conundrum of an illogical and devastating dental schedule, but I decided to give it the old college try anyway (and I went to two of them)! Looking back, the straw that had broken my hump came on an unremarkable yet fateful Wednesday when I noticed that I had seven crown preparations to execute, on seven different patients. Are you kidding me? That was a lot of work to do and I would certainly run behind all day. Who created this looming disaster? It was a mess and not a masterpiece of masterful scheduling! I exploded and blew my top. But the responsible front office staff wouldn't have it. They quietly and reassuringly told me that I had wanted to be more productive, so they were just carrying out my orders. What? Did I really say that? Maybe I did, come to think of it. Darn it. Perhaps I was my own worst enemy? I just barely made it through that day and then lashed out at everyone in earshot. But before I thankfully left for home, I uncharacteristically ordered a mandatory lunchtime staff meeting Taco Pronto! The next day I bought "food" from Taco Bell and we hashed it out for an hour straight in the waiting room while noshing on double-burrito-stuffed chimichangas jammed into chalupas and rolled up inside giant enchiladas. Quixotically, I began whining about my workload while praising the money being generated by the practice. The seven-member female staff complained about me complaining all the time, but what else was new? I glanced at the ticking wall clock and realized we had five

138

minutes left to address the actual scheduling situation and we finally did, with one minute to spare before the afternoon's first victim arrived. I did most of the hurried speaking and quickly yelled out the following gems: As the latest continuing education seminars and dental journal articles so poignantly pointed out, the office members and not the patients should run the asylum. Duh! Firstly, WE were in charge and needed to retrain everyone, including ourselves. Secondly, patients would be put in the "book" for maximum daily productivity, namely, big cases in the morning when I was fresh (I was always a little fresh), followed by little ones in the afternoon. It was scientifically called Block Scheduling, for maximum dental production. Unfortunately, my crack (more like cracked) staff had always thought the phrase was blockhead scheduling, because that's how they currently and haphazardly appointed patients. And thirdly, emergency patients would have certain chunks of time specifically reserved for them and could no longer come in willy-nilly as shoehorned side-books. We were all excited to launch our new, improved and streamlined front office protocols. However, in a few weeks time I covertly evaluated our progress, or lack thereof. Unfortunately, we were reverting to old patterns and habits once more and I could feel that toxic, overwrought, and tense feeling returning to the office.

What had gone wrong? The patients, who else? Not everyone could come in as orchestrated. Not everyone could leave their jobs at specific times to be accommodated for toothaches, either. The careful choreography of shuffling humans around for our own monetary and mental benefits had failed. We tried and sort of got some of it right, but in the end I had to lace up the old roller-skates once more if I wanted to stay busy and appease my clientele. The winners were the patients; I was the big loser. Of course success can be measured in different ways, such as income earned and gratefully witnessing the growth of a practice. Nevertheless, and as Tölle had mentioned, I sure wanted to run away on many a day and still do at times.

24

Doggonit

What did I look like, a puzzle master? Evidently yes as widowed Mrs. Blackman dejectedly sat down in the dental chair and tearfully unburdened her story. But wait a minute; didn't I recently deliver a magnificent upper denture to her, one that she just loved to pieces? Yes, it was the same Mrs. Blackman who now handed over to me a Ziploc bag filled with fractured denture pieces. She was distraught and inconsolable. "Could you please put my plate back together again?" she cried as I carefully counted out thirty broken chunks of pink acrylic/white teeth on the sterile countertop next to me. Then I told her flat out that I could not glue her denture back together into a Frankenstein-like prosthesis. "It just wouldn't fit or look the same," I cautioned. "But I loved them so much," she blubbered. "How did this happen?" I quizzically asked. "Did you drink some HARD cider?" I further quipped, trying to lighten the mood in the operatory. "No, my Lab did it," she murmured. "Now, my lab makes things; it doesn't break them," I joked, and that elicited a slight smile from her. Good, at least the tears had stopped, and we could finally get to the bottom of things and move on. And then she told me her tale, or tail, I should say. Mr. Bojangles, Mrs. Blackman's black, one-year-old, Labrador retriever was a large and feisty adolescent canine. She related that he was constantly in motion and curious about a great many things – kind of like a cat. And she would always catch him excitedly nosing around her personal possessions and dancing a lick in pure pleasure whenever he found something to play with. It turns out that one night as she dosed off in her favorite armchair, while watching *Dancing with the Stars*, her mouth fell open and Mr. Bojangles noticed. He carefully crept up to the sofa, put both paws on the arms of the chair, leaned in and ever so gently removed the upper denture from her mouth. That's what she said, anyway. My eyes grew wide as I listened intently. Her story was gripping. All of a sudden, she awoke to happy whimpering and crunching noises near her. Although in a groggy state, she claimed that she looked down at her feet and witnessed her daffy dog blissfully destroying her choppers. And by the time she fully regained her faculties and shooed him away it was just too late. And then she started to bawl while seeing the chewed remnants that were scattered on her black, bearskin rug. She yelled at him as he went cowering into a corner as she sadly gathered up the evidence. Bad dog, for sure! Unfortunately, dogs can be like that. Even more unfortunate was Mr. Bojangles' cunning and stealthy removal and subsequent massacre of Mrs. Blackman's denture in the first place. What a sneak he was. Anyway, I fabricated a new upper denture for her, and I recall charging her half price for the prosthesis. Once more she left the office smiling and promised not to let Mr. Bojangles anywhere near her cake hole. Good thinking, I guess. I just hope she quickly let him in on the new set of rules in HIS roost.

25

Crimes and Punishments

This is a sordid tale involving two formerly delightful patients who I mistakenly thought were my friends. Inexplicably, both ended up turning against me, each in a most peculiar way (shout-out to David Bowie!). Each one had lulled me into a false sense of security, then WHAM! Anyway, I had been actively perusing dentate literature in the late '90s and enthusiastically followed the dental dogma of the day, namely, if you wanted a patient's loyalty, you had to truly befriend her/him. And not in a phony, patronizing way but in a sincere and empathetic manner that really showed how much you cared. Nevertheless, I'm sure that dentists born with a clever tongue had it easier than some others. I did alright but it all seemed like a contrived dalliance, and were dentists just looking for trouble? Here goes…. B.B. worked for the State and had GHI dental insurance (one of the lowest of the low), which I took as full payment. That was the arrangement; there were no out-of-pocket co-pays for the patient. As a dental provider either you fully participated with GHI or you did not. B.B. was a middle-aged, stout blabbermouth and an ingratiating kind of woman, the kind that made friends easily. And she carried that tradition into my office, notwithstanding the dental disaster she presented me with. However, B.B. seemed to take her flaky dentition in stride and frequently boasted: "My mouth has always been a sinking wreck." We both laughed easily at that canard and I became ENTRUSTED to steer her listing oral ship. I had unwittingly yet voluntarily inherited her toothy troubles from a previous dentist whom she would not mention. We instantly set up a positive rapport and she confided in me that she wished to stop drinking and chain smoking, too. She TRUSTED me with her confidences, and I was elated to gain a dental pal. But besides a few cavities to be filled, her real dental dilemma was advanced periodontal disease. Although her teeth were firm, the gradual loss of bone anchoring them would lead to their eventual loss. Her deleterious smoking (mainly chain-smoking unfiltered Camels) and imbibing habits were probably partly to blame for her oral disposition as well. I had initially recognized her disastrous dentition and vigorously pushed for her to see a gum specialist, even noting our discussion in her hand-written chart. However, periodontists in our area did not take any type of dental insurances so that avenue of redress was quickly dismissed by her. She flatly stated that she did not have four grand to spend on a specialist, period. So, years went by with my hygienists regularly cleaning her teeth, taking routine radiographs and me supervising her ongoing neglect by limited documentation. At that point, what was the point of reading her the riot act? She had been coming to my office for years, seemed content in her running diagnosis of a gradually failing dentition, and kept up her bon vivant mannerisms with my staff and me. We small-talked about our vacations, politics, the weather, etc. She was a great gal, or was she? One day she came in as an emergency patient for a lower left molar (number 19) which had suddenly become very mobile and painful (active periodontal disease can be episodic and random). Even though her mouth stunk of stale cigarette smoke and liquor, I was polite and jovial around her as usual. I recommended her to see one of my favorite oral surgeons for the extraction, gave her a prescription for an antibiotic and sent her on her way. And for a long while I heard nothing. Not that I was a nosy *nudnik* and pining for a reply from her, but at the very least a post-surgical treatment note from the oral surgeon would have been nice. However, nothing. And then THE LETTER came and my heart more than sank. I felt the knife plunge deep into my left ventricle! I was to appear at a deposition hearing involving B.B. and a locally famous dental malpractice attorney which she had hired. What? And for what? I was more than stunned. My staff could see

the color drained from my face and realized I was in some
sort of major legal jeopardy. Holy shit! And of all people,
B.B.! What did I ever do to her? Maybe it was for what I
didn't do but should have done? All kinds of thoughts were
zinging around my brain as I secured my liability
insurance-appointed council, B.B.'s voluminous records
and her large pile of mounted x-rays. I met with my
assigned attorney and he assured me that based on my
sheer volume of paperwork and notations, I should be in
good shape to win the evidentiary day and not go to trial.
He and I met at the opposing lawyer's posh office and I
immediately sensed something wrong. What were B.B.'s
husband and young son doing there? And why were all
three of them crying profusely, wiping their tears away and
blowing noses ad nauseum? I was being set up, but why? I
glared at B.B. across the large wooden oak table and she
glared right back at me. After the initial introductions and
after the waterworks had ceased from the other side, I got
kicked in the head by the plaintiff's plainspoken, frumpy,
yet highfalutin-acting counselor. B.B.'s attorney boiled it
down rather succinctly for me: The oral surgeon had
somehow convinced her that instead of an extraction, she
should seek immediate treatment with a periodontist. And
since my notes made no mention of that fact for many
years, I was beyond negligent and had misguided and

147

grossly misled poor B.B. into the dental state she was now in. "I TRUSTED you!" B.B. blubbered out loud as her husband and son started to bawl again as if to reinforce the fact that I had ruined all their lives and not just hers. That really hurt. I sat back and knew this was not going to end well. And it didn't. My visibly agitated lawyer vainly tried to present my side of things, stating that the patient had basically abrogated any responsibility for her failing dentition and did not wish to see a periodontist. Her lawyer was unmoved and said that based on my "uncaring attitude," scant records and lack of a patient-signed periodontal consent form releasing me from liability, a court would find me guilty of all kinds of dental abuses. And he should know; he was the local kingpin of the courts. WTF? What should I have done differently? Physically kidnapped her and then deposited her at a periodontal office and paid for any treatment out my own pocket? Is that what friends were for? I was simultaneously angry and depressed. After listening to some more threatening jargon from the opposition, my side caved. My attorney whispered to me that it was better to make a deal now than risk a trial. So he did just that. The whole affair was settled for five grand, which included her lawyer's fee. My insurance company would cough up the dough and my annual premium would take a steep hike, but it was now over. Now she could afford a gum specialist and "properly save" her teeth. However, they were unsavable, even by an expert. Unless she quit her damaging vices and magically regrew bone in her jaws, any surgical or grafting intervention would be futile. Even I knew that, and I was not a gum specialist. Nevertheless, she got the *gelt* and I got the gate. And that's how you effectively end a dental friendship! However, I still did not learn my lesson. Three years hence, in 1999, something similar transpired. Mr. Grober was a large, garrulous man and had worked for the State in an upper echelon position for years. He claimed to know everyone there. He too had the bottom-of-the-barrel GHI dental insurance plan, found my office, and became a regular patron for years. And he was also a lot of fun. Always quick with a joke for all within earshot, he was a pleasure to see and work on. Our "sketch comedy routine" was such that he would loudly ask me if the shot would hurt and I would always reply, "No, it won't hurt me a bit, but thanks for asking!" That punch line elicited much tittering and sometimes outright laughter from the staff and patients who overheard our boisterous conversations. HIPAA be damned! It was all part of the gag, our unique dental bonding *shtick* that we had established between ourselves. He was my friend, or was he? After completing most of his restorative dental work over the years, such as a

149

few crowns and many fillings, only a lower right, three-unit bridge remained to be fabricated. No sweat, right? Wrong! The bridge was a bear to do. The back molar was so badly broken down that I had to prepare the tooth well below the gumline. Nevertheless, I was used to working in difficult situations, after all, I was a trained prosthodontist and experienced in such matters. But the deep decay had somehow managed to confound me, nonetheless. The final impressions and temporary bridge were made, and the "happy" patient was dismissed. Two weeks later Mr. Grober came back in with a broken temporary bridge, but no matter. I was going to cement in the permanent one that day anyhow. We bantered, we *kibitzed* noisily and then I seated the bridge in place. However, before permanently cementing it I had my dental assistant snap an x-ray of it, to make sure it fit well. I did not always do this with all my prosthetic dentistry but felt that I should in this case. And my fears were realized. I saw the blatantly obvious open bridge margin at the base of the molar that I had trouble with earlier. In all good conscience and adhering to proper dental ethics, I could not and would not glue that bridge in place. But no biggie. I nonchalantly told the patient that we had to remake it at no charge and that things would work out. No problem. Easy breezy. Ha. However, Mr. Grober anxiously spoke up and stated that he had to go out of town for a few weeks and reminded me that his previous temporary bridge had cracked in half and disintegrated. He begged me to permanently affix the final bridge. I said no, not with permanent cement. However, I could put it in with temporary cement with one proviso: that he had to return right after his trip for me to redo the job and make things right. We were on very friendly terms, so I wasn't worried about any dental fallout. And there should not have been any. I waved good-bye to him as he left. "Okie dokie, Doc.," he yelled upon exiting and that was the last time I ever saw him. And then I received THAT LETTER; the one that could make your blood curdle. But this time it was not from a lawyer's office but from OPD, the Office of Professional Discipline. This office was part of the state education department and could suspend or revoke a dental license. These were the bad boys, the ones you did not want to cross. As I read the short letter, there was Mr. Grober's name attached to it! What the hell? I know he worked in the same building as OPD but why did he get THEM involved? There was no reason to. I thought he liked me? Fast forward a few weeks and there I meekly sat, alongside the provided defense attorney from my malpractice carrier, and listened passively to the three, very elderly and wizened dental adjudicators who could seal my professional fate in a heartbeat. They reviewed everything first, like to make sure I was actually a dentist, etc. They also became slightly annoyed that I was a prosthodontic specialist and had made Mr. Grober sign the usual treatment consent form. I was hot, testy and sweaty and tried to answer their inane questions in an even tone. My attorney just sat there stone-faced and said nothing. Finally, after reviewing the patient's x-rays and records, and after taking into account my side of the fiasco, I was told to wait outside while they decided my dental fate. Those ten minutes felt like hours and I maddeningly paced the hallway but not before looking around and seeing at least twenty dour and defeated-looking dentists and their respective lawyers, all nervously sitting on metal chairs, waiting to be called in after me. This "crime and punishment gig" was a fulltime racket for the State! Who knew? And who knew that there were so many shitty dentists out there who needed to be disciplined? But more importantly, how did I end up being one of them? My council called me back inside and I was found guilty – of having incomplete records. I protested and started to say that I could not write a novel during every patient encounter, but my lawyer wisely kicked me hard under the table and I shut my sarcastic trap. The head honcho said that while I was innocent of willful wrongdoing, I had wasted their precious time and they had to get me on something. Huh? What about MY time and MY piece of mind? I was fined $500.00 for poor record keeping and laughed out of the OPD office. My attorney vigorously shook my hand in a victory squeeze and told me that I had done great. But wait. Was OPD just a money-making machine for the State, to shake down dentists based on allegations and flimsy proof? I did not know and was still puzzled as to how I had gotten into this predicament in the first place. So instead of leaving, I marched right back into that den of despair and confronted all three dentists before the next hapless sap took the hot seat. It was unprecedented, unforeseen and threw them for a loop. They cowered in a neutral corner as if I was going to physically pummel them. Maybe my angry countenance and athletic physique had scared them? I had secretly hoped so. Anyway, all I wanted to know was who had blown the whistle and ratted me out, and why? And they surprisingly and obligingly spilled the beans. It turned out that Mr. Grober had consulted another local dentist prior to leaving on his trip because the provisionally cemented permanent bridge had fallen out. That dentist, in addition to also temporarily cementing the bridge, had verbally thrown me under the bus. He had dismissively called my work shoddy and sloppy. As to why Mr. Grober had not returned to me for his emergency avulsion is a mystery.

Perhaps he was embarrassed for losing the bridge so soon? I don't know. In any event, the new dentist had permanently poisoned any residual goodwill that Mr. Grober harbored toward me and encouraged him to punish yours truly. And it wasn't even about the money, which I gladly would have given back. It was the vindictive vitriol that the new dentist had purposely implanted in Mr. Grober which had done me in. And that really chafed me. We all knew about those sell-out dentists who routinely criticized other dentists' work. They embraced that hundred-year-old pizza box slogan that proclaims, "You've tried the rest, now try the best!" Really? Did their shit not stink? We were told in dental school never to demean other dentists' therapies because we were not in their shoes when said dental work occurred. However, some irascible and pompous pricks got the message yet decided they were above the fray of mediocrity and fancied themselves as the saviors of dentistry. Give me a break. And their ilk is still around, I'm afraid. However, I was not out of the woods quite yet. Mr. Grober could have sued me for malpractice as well and did not. Nor did he take me to small claims court to at least get the insurance money back. Perhaps my punishment by a governing dental body was enough for him? Thankfully, it was. Anyway, in conclusion, I would like to extend a thank you to all the dentists out there who have eyeballed my treatments up close and never disparaged them, even out of spite. And I'm sure I have had a lot of close calls with self-righteous dentists over my nearly four-decade career; dentists who wanted to pull the trigger on me but did not. Thank you! But the same holds true for me. Oftentimes I will shake my head but offer no condemning verbiage upon seeing inadequate or dilapidated dentistry from a previous dentist. It is better to tactfully explain the situation to the patient and not to belittle anything or anyone. Unless of course that dentist happens to be one of THOSE aforementioned, hated shills and had it coming to him/her!

26

Beware the Old Bag

Not quite one score into this so-called dental *shtick* and I was being burned by unscrupulous patients less and less. It was experience plus developing a cynically savvy attitude: namely that not every situation encountered was necessarily on the up and up. It was depressing to constantly be vigilant for possible psychological shenanigans and open hostilities which could occur at any time. But that was how the dental game was unfolding for me and, like a *putz* in a "nice guy" recovery program, I took it one day at a time. Stooped and gray, Mrs. Ridgelap presented herself at my posh, boutique-like, prosthodontic practice, the one I started from scratch in a sophisticated city after selling my hurried and insurance-driven nightmare in Milfton Park. She had come on the recommendation of a close friend who raved about my purposely slow-paced office, giant saltwater fish tank, and excellent dental services. So far, so good. "What can I do you for, Mrs. Ridgelap?" I jokingly asked her; intentionally mixing up the syntax of my question just for a bit of fun. "Well," she began, "I need new teeth, Doctor, and you are the man I was told to see." Again, so far, so good. However, as I was carefully examining her edentulous mouth, with the soothing sounds of Nora Jones wafting from the office CD player, I couldn't help but notice Mrs. Ridgelap clutching a small, tattered, brown paper bag. I motioned to my dental assistant R. who gently asked if her lunch was in it? It was a throw-away query just to be friendly and Mrs. Ridgelap did not take umbrage. She happily proceeded to open it for me. I looked inside and counted maybe eight or nine dentures. She had no chompers in her mouth and then frankly proceeded to lambast previous dentists for their combined incompetence and her resultant dire straits. "I don't have a decent set of plates," she wailed. I suddenly "smelled a rat" and those proverbial warning bells went off in my skull. I leaned back in my dentist's chair and before starting any dental conversation thought back to 1985, my third year in dental school. In my Removable Prosthodontics clinic Dr. Sherman, a favorite professor of mine, once told me in a Flatbush-Sheepshead Bay-Yiddish accent, "Beware of an old bag carrying an old bag full of dentures. There is no way in Hell that ALL of her former dentists were *schlubs*!" "Mayputz," he affectionately growled, "Don't be the fifth or sixth fool in an old bag." I got the message from wise old Dr. Sherman and remember it to this day. Sometimes a new set of oral prostheses just doesn't work out, regardless of the effort put in by the dentist or the desires of the willing patient. Deleterious reasons can include inadequate underlying jawbone support to a heightened gag reflex. There does not have to be anything nefarious going on, sometimes bad luck is all it is, but I did not want to be any part of it. So far, not so good. Anyhow, I cleared my head of the momentary mnemonic and professionally explained to Mrs. Ridgelap why I could not undertake the fabrication of her dentures. She started to protest and mentioned her friend, but it was all in vain. I told her that I did not feel brave enough embarking on this project after so many good doctors had failed before me. Once again she raised her voice in displeasure at my seemingly glib response. "Don't you want my money?" was her last-ditch pitch to me. "No, it's not that. I believe the dental gods will not favor me while I'm working on you," I replied, only in half jest. She grinned awkwardly but seemed to accept that lame answer in resignation. She knew I would not treat her. In truth, once I lost confidence in a dental case, it was hard for me to jump back in for "the old college try." Mrs. Ridgelap gathered herself, closed her weathered paper bag and left on her own volition. I had not even charged her a consultation fee. And she didn't leave in anger but in dismay. However, in the immortal words of lifelong Brooklynite Dr. Sherman: "Beware the old bag. And if she won't leave voluntarily, give that old bag the sack!" That guy was a real pip and I miss him. I'm sure he had dental stories galore that would make mine seem "bush league" in comparison.

27

Kitty's Plaything

Miss Kitka, a calico cat probably named after the Catwoman's alter ego character in the '60s *Batman* TV show, was just a playful kitten according to her elderly owner Miss Graboobner. Lots of family and friends would come over to her house and invariably bring a new cat-toy for Miss Kitka to play with. And, as per her owner, there was nothing inherently special about the indoor cat except for a penchant for playing long and hard with her playthings. Be it stringed, catnip-stuffed or rodent-resembling objects, Miss Kitka loved them all. So there didn't seem to be anything out of the ordinary as Miss Graboobner watched her kitty-cat having fun on the floor one day. "She has a bunch of shiny knickknacks that she likes to paw, scratch and bite," said the lady to me in a low tone. I struggled to hear her when she suddenly bellowed, "And then I realized that the damn cat was wrestling with my lower plate! I thought it was one of those silvery "fishing lures" for cats that one of my kids had bought her but, no, it was my fuckin' partial denture, Doc. I had left it by the bathroom sink after cleaning it and forgot to stick it back in my mouth." I was stunned not only at her loud outburst and curse word usage but at the audacity of a supposedly well-fed and loved feline to be so emboldened as to "mess" with her owner. But then I thought of my own deceased but beloved cats, Skyler and Sherman. They too tried my patience when they seemingly willfully misbehaved. But they were cats and that's what cats do! They tip over vases for no apparent reason, investigate any "new" space or hiding places, jump into boxes, scatter and rip up a newspaper before you finish reading it, and routinely demonstrate an ambivalent and lackadaisical love for their human owners. Cats. What else can I say? "Miss Graboobner, I think your cat is a real *trip*," I jokingly said. Miss Graboobner would have none of it and tartly replied, "Don't say nice things about my pussy, because you've never seen her." Fair enough, I shut my trap. I ended up making Miss Graboobner a new partial lower prosthesis because she insisted on it, even though the slightly chewed and bent one might have still fit her mouth. And she also insisted on paying me full fare because it was the fault of her prized pet. That Miss Kitka; I could have used a crafty cat like that to drum up business with. Perhaps I could have loaned her out to my patients' homes to do some dirty work for me. You know, create havoc and mischief with any oral appliances left lying around. If only cats could be trained in that way. Oh, well; I shouldn't be having thoughts like that, should I?

28

Fighting Entropy

"I can't believe YOUR bridge broke," exclaimed the elderly and perfectly coiffed woman in an accusatory tone. I abruptly sat back in my dentist's chair and stared at her. Oh, nice; some greeting, right from the get-go! I hadn't even said hello, yet. Nevertheless, upon closer examination, her face DID look familiar; I just didn't know where to put it. Then I saw a jaundiced name on the newly made-up chart and unfortunately recollected her. "Mrs. Disser," I slowly began, "When did we make this bridge?" "Twenty years ago, to be exact, Doctor Mayputz," she spurted out. I had not seen this lady for two decades, yet she hunted me down just to show me the alleged calamity in her cakehole? Why not have her current dentist take care of it? Did she think she had a written lifetime warranty with me? What the hell? I had never signed such a document with anyone. I didn't know if such a thing even existed in other dental practices. Most current cars will only give you a three-year bumper to bumper deal. Why should dentistry be any different? Oh, sure, I had replaced faulty prostheses for free or only for the lab bill if they were a few years old, or if the laboratory work was positively deemed inadequate. My compassionate scruples were virtuous for the most part. But this was a first for me. Did she just want to rub it in my face, or did she really want me to replace that bridge with a new one after all these years? "I have fillings and gold crowns that are older than this crappy bridge," she crassly crowed, further rubbing salt into my wounded dental pride. A detailed inspection of her dentition revealed a few places where porcelain had indeed chipped off the four-unit fixed bridge, yet the metal understructure and marginal fits were intact, and the bite was fully functional. The small deficits were not in a cosmetic zone and only her tongue could detect them. What the eff? I told her I could quickly smooth off the rough spots and that the bridge was still OK. She stared at me long and hard with a disbelieving countenance on her twisted mug. "You mean I came all the way up here just so you could sand down your work of art?" she sarcastically snarled. However, I did just that, did not charge her, and emphatically told her that twenty years was a long time for anything to last. She didn't buy it and threatened to sue me as she left in a huff. At this point I had heard many bluffs of litigation from unhappy campers. So I chose not to let her diatribe get my dandruff up. A younger Dr. Mayputz would have apologized profusely or tried to assuage her in a genuflecting way. Perhaps that's what she was really after, watching me squirm while she gleefully confirmed my supposed ineptitude? Unfortunately, my burned out and beaten-up ego was in no mood to kowtow to yet another asshole looking for vengeful rectitude. Then I thought about the whole situation some more. What in the universe gets better or more orderly with the passage of time? Nothing. A loose interpretation of the word entropy tells us that things in life tend toward disorder, no matter how much we try not to let that happen. Things wear out in time and objects break, etc. After thousands of masticatory cycles, what did patients expect from artificially placed pieces of ceramic in their mouths? Can any dentist really deliver the goods for a lengthy lifetime of chewing? I don't think so. Am I also to be held responsible for patients who eat rocks or open beer bottles with their pearly fangs? Is that what Mrs. Disser was doing? Who knows; patients lie to me all the time. And remember, dental insurance companies will usually cover their portion of the expense to replace a crown or bridge after a five to ten-year period of service. Their algorithms predict failure way before twenty years! Entropy is the key word here Mrs. Disser, so piss off. Fortuitously, I never got a legal summons in the mail or ANY feedback from her. I hope her current dentist has a cast iron stomach lining and fabricates any future prosthetic devices for her out of solid metal. It might just last her a lifetime.

29

Nice Guys Finish Last

That title does not refer to a woman's preference when coupling with a male paramour, although it probably should. No, it is most often used as a facetious euphemism to describe failure in life due to being a wimpy wussy, or something along that line. The business world, including dentistry, is seemingly replete with examples where celebrated traits such as shrewdness and cunning supersede sympathy and empathy. Not only does the early bird get the worm but the clever and back-stabbing bird also gets the worm and a whole lot more! Anyhow, elderly and ever so polite Mrs. Cockburn had been coming to my swanky, prosthodontic, boutique practice for some time now. It was the practice I had started from scratch after selling my previous one. In this iteration, I only had one well-paid female employee, who doubled as a receptionist and assistant. The fee-for-service office was small and cozy and had all the trappings and comforts of a spa. Plus, I had outfitted it with the latest state-of-the-art dental equipment as well. It was a soothing place to patronize and Mrs. Cockburn loved coming to her appointments. That's what she told me, anyway. I ended up replacing a few of her faulty fillings and conservatively repaired some fractured teeth yet during every appointment she would invariably bring up the topic of the symmetrical spaces she had on either side of her lower dentition. However, every time I would bring up the price of dual fixed bridges, she would say, "I love you Dr. Mayputz, but not that much." We both chuckled at that sarcastic sentiment and nothing was ever done about those missing teeth. I could have made a partial denture, but she insisted on having permanent and not removable prosthetic teeth. One day my dental assistant told me that Mrs. Cockburn was coming in as an emergency patient because one of her ancient front fillings had popped out. I relished the thought of interacting with that old dame because she was fun and always squared up at the end. So imagine my unbelievable shock when I examined her mouth and saw that those bilateral lower spaces had been closed with two bridges, only I did not fabricate them! What the hell? I immediately questioned her about the fiasco in her oral cavity. "Well, I only went to him because my neighbor told me to," she spat out. "And then he gave me a little blue pill and when I woke up, I had these two bridges in my mouth," she indignantly added. I'm the one who should have been indignant, not her! She made it sound like she went to another dental office under duress and was forced at gunpoint to get dental work done. Give me a break. And about that little blue pill – I assumed it was a common short-acting tranquilizer called Halcion .25mg and not a Viagra tablet, which is similar in shape and color. But perhaps it WAS a Viagra pill and she suddenly got horny for bridges? It was a funny thought but even I wasn't laughing. Nonetheless, who was this interloper dentist and where was his office? Didn't she tell him she was my longtime patient? Maybe he didn't care? On top of that he charged her more than I would have and got away with it. And here she was complaining intimately to me as if I was her son, instead of an unrelated dental professional. I was steamed yet Mrs. Cockburn did not seem to grasp the depth of my anger or bewilderment. Then my dental assistant piped in and told me, in front of her, that she knew of a dentist over on Broadway who "specialized" in sedation dentistry, had a reputation for being disreputable, and was a bit of an aggressive con man. It sounded like he specialized in mining for gold in patients' wallets! Evidently, rumor had it that he zonked people out and when they awoke, would have more dentistry in their respective mouths than they had agreed to before treatment commenced. Was he a crafty and diabolical dweeb in his dental school days as well? "Did he get rich because of those same abject and ruthless behaviors, now skillfully employed on his unwary and naïve patients," I rhetorically murmured to myself? Some things never change. Mrs. Cockburn seemed to nod in agreement and sighed as if she was deeply wronged. Then she stated that I was much nicer than he and she would continue to see me from now on. Yeah, I really trusted her now; her word was good – Not! Yet upon reflection Mrs. Cockburn might have been confused or mistaken when signing multiple consent forms in his office? Or maybe he really was a fast-talking dental slickster and got away with pulling underhanded shit all the time. Who knows? However, I was still mad, because HE got the dough, and I was the *schmo*! I hated being taken advantage of in that manner and basically stopped treating her after that episode. Perhaps it wasn't completely her fault and I overreacted? Maybe. But any way you sliced it I ended up being the patsy, a nice guy that finished dead last, at least in the dental sweepstakes called Mrs. Cockburn.

30

Back to Back

When it rains, it pours, or so "they" say. I had two litigious actions brought against me within a one month span causing my longtime professional dental liability (malpractice) insurance company to seriously question its relationship with me. You know, whether or not to drop me like a hot potato for supposedly being a bad risk. However, it had a valid reason to be so concerned: it has to stay profitable in order to pay out a few paltry claims at the top while sucking in bushels of Benjamins from the bottom. Kind of how a water fountain or a "legal" Ponzi scheme works, but that's basically how all insurances operate. I hoped they would not can me, and they ultimately did not. Whew. Anyway, it had been a long legal, dry spell for me, approximately ten years since my last brush with the law, either good or bad. And as per usual, first came the dreaded, gold-embossed-with-raised-lettering, lawyerly, envelope which indubitably signaled a potential heart attack for the addressee upon opening. I ripped it apart and quickly scanned the gorgeous letterhead and that one paragraph of doom as my anxiety and pulse rate hit the ceiling. I was to be summoned to a local court of law on behest of a disgruntled female patient. That part was evident, but this was not a small-claims-court matter and who the hell was she, anyway? I quickly tried to recall all the recent "troublemaking patients" that are part of most dental practices; the ones who you figure will sue you at the drop of a hat. But, no, I didn't readily recognize the name as I grabbed her thinly papered chart and began reading my notes. Now I remembered. She was the "bag lady" referred to me by a local general dentist to restore an implant which he could not. I charged her a very nominal consultation fee, had taken only one x-ray and deemed the implant non-restorable. Her occlusion had collapsed to the point that the implant could not have a crown routinely affixed to it without first raising her entire bite with expensive and drawn-out dentistry. It was all clearly documented by me in her notes and I was puzzled as to her cause of claim. I recalled telling her that I was a prosthodontist and not a magician; sometimes oral conditions could not be easily ameliorated. She in turn told me that she had no "big" money and seemed to have understood that a single restorative procedure could not be promptly accomplished. She still had remaining teeth and could chew, so it was never a case of me being a cold lout and refusing to treat a shabby "hobo" with a perceived lack of funds. She packed up her bags and scuttled out of my office to go back to the referring dentist. In other words, I could not help her, but neither could he. But how could she afford a lawyer, I wondered? Was it her cousin Vinnie? The lawyer's first name on the letterhead was Vincent, by the way. Anyhow, I quickly phoned my malpractice carrier, was given a defense attorney and was ready to appear in front of a judge. My assigned council had me send him the patient records and then expressed bewilderment at the merits of the suit. He was puzzled as to why I was dragged into this after not having rendered any treatment at all. He was somewhat confused when we met in person, about an hour before it was my turn in the docket. And wait; there was the referring general dentist and his lawyer as well. We were all there, including my dental assistant, standing around inside the spacious foyer and nervously bantering small talk before being ushered into the vacuous county courthouse. Finally it was our turn. My attorney was clutching copies of my patient's paperwork and I had the originals in hand as we reverently took our seats in the front pew. And then the monkeyshines began! For the next hour or so, the perplexed judge was treated to an apoplectic woman who repeatedly shushed her own council, and who wove a woeful tale so incredible that my mouth remained open the whole time. Nebulous and far-reaching collusion theories were vehemently launched by her; namely, that the

171

referring dentist and I conspired to deny her adequate dental care. With arms flailing amid a myriad of rustling papers, she would have made Perry Mason proud. She was that good at presenting a case of malfeasance, misconduct and malpractice against the referring dentist and me. She also insinuated that I was not a real specialist and should be severely punished with a lengthy prison term for impersonating a prosthodontist. Was she a former or current lawyer herself? Did she attend a low ranked and chintzy college such as Albany Law School back in the day and now spouted off legalese out of spite? Maybe. But I felt guilty just listening to her and then the disbelieving judge spoke up, after interviewing us two dentists and carefully studying all the pertinent materials offered. "Why are you here, lady? You have no case. Both dentists have stated under oath that they cannot restore your mouth to proper form and function without a significant outlay of time and money which you have stated that you do not have. Neither dentist has performed negligent or iatrogenic dentistry in your mouth. The dental diagnostic fees charged were reasonable and you are free to consult other dentists if you so desire. Case dismissed," he emphatically summed up while nearly driving his gavel through the desktop. Then there was a prolonged moment of silence. I didn't know whether to laugh or cry. My attorney, who had basically said two words during the "Big Show," smiled at me, at the judge and then packed up to leave. The judge grinned back as we defense parties stared at the plaintiff and her legal beagle in anticipation of a last and furtive, insulting salvo. But none came. She picked up all her strewn-about papers, muttered some type of obscenity, which the judge heard but ignored, and slowly shuffled out of the building with her lawyer in tow. My sweaty palms slowly dried as the judge uncharacteristically turned to me and the other dentist and apologized on behalf of himself and the good people of the county. Thanks Judgy-Wudgy, you were a real pal. My dental assistant, my lawyer and I vacated the court, but I still did not know why I had been forced to appear there in the first place. It wasn't about the money. It seemed to have been about an aggrieved patient who mistakenly thought she was dentally abused by two uncaring and "wealthy" dentists and then thought it was her civic duty to expose us "charlatans" for the good of society. Was that it? She had wanted her day in court, and she got it. Fuck a duck! The next situation I unfortunately became embroiled in had to do with gum disease. The elderly and quirky patient had recently moved to the area from New Jersey and just happened to chance upon my office due to a recommendation from a new neighbor. Although a prosthodontic specialist, I still saw many general dental patients in my practice. So, Mr. Pisspotte came in and had no sooner sat down before he started to regale me with adulating stories about his previous dentist. He had been a longtime patient of this doctor and idolized him. He then said that he hoped and prayed that I could live up to the lofty standard of excellence set by that Jersey dentist. "Wow, I have my work cut out for me if I'm going to please this rude dude," I thought to myself. And then the big reveal: a potty mouth awash with puffy, inflamed gingiva and in desperate need of restorative repair. What the hell? And to confirm my suspicions based on the oral and radiographic evidence, I gently and deliberately probed ALL the spaces between his teeth and gums and had my dental assistant write down the values in indelible black ink. This loquacious bloke had seriously advanced periodontal disease and it was my doctorly and ethical duty to inform him. Or was it? I restudied his x-rays and pointed out the need for many fillings. He was okay with that but when I matter-of-factly mentioned a major problem with his gum tissues, he went ballistic and started cussing loudly. And when I interjected that he needed to see a periodontist, or at the very least have me initiate a deep cleaning, Mr. Pisspotte went nuclear. "You are so full of shit, Doc," he angrily chimed in, and then added, "My dentist was the greatest, you are a nobody. I am out of here, you money-grubbing asswipe!" And with that he tore off his patient bib, tossed it on the floor and stomped out of the office without so much as making a payment or offering a deferential goodbye. My dental assistant and I just stood there looking at each other in amazement but then laughed it off as yet another "crazy" whom we would never hear from again. I documented my dental findings as well as the patient/doctor verbal altercation while chuckling the whole time. That guy was a real piece of work! Ha, ha. However, a few weeks later, I was not the one laughing. There was THAT envelope again, the kind I hated to open: the one with an attorney's return address on it. Crap! Now who wanted a piece of me? Once more I thought of all my disgruntled patients who could possibly have it out for me and wondered aloud. Who could it be this time and so soon, too? I just had a recent outing with the law, and now again? Two cases in one month. Damn! With my neck hairs standing on end, I read the enclosed parchment. That catty cad from New Jersey was the one taking me to court for malpractice, mental injury and for insulting his previous dentist! What? I hadn't done anything to him, or for him. I had only seen him once to deliver a dire diagnosis, and that's all. And the fucker still owed me money. WTF? My stalwart dental assistant, the same insurance lawyer that had represented me before, and

I slowly trudged up the steps of the same courthouse, took seats in the back row and waited for the showdown. The plaintiff showed up on time and sat down at the other end of the spacious room. But where was his attorney? I surmised that anyone could bring a lawsuit against anyone if they were perseverant and knew what paperwork to file and with whom. I looked up and there was the same judge that had adjudicated my prior suit and I breathed a sigh of relief. I hoped that he remembered me and his previous judgment in my favor. As my party and I approached the bench for our turn he looked benevolently upon me and smiled, then grimaced at the dour patient. Mr. Pisspotte excitedly began his spiel but after ten minutes of wildly gesturing and arguing nonsense, the judge cut him off and said that he had heard enough. Then he cleared his throat and growled, "So, what you are saying is that Dr. Mayputz, a well-respected dental specialist in town, is guilty of 'finding' and diagnosing periodontal disease in your mouth out of the blue whereas your previous godly dentist had never mentioned it? Is that correct?" "Yes," said the lawyer-less patient who stood up to continue his jabbering rant. "Sit down," warned the stern judge, and then added, "And you are further alleging that Dr. Mayputz is incompetent and only out for his best interests and not yours? Correct? And you have proof of his malpractice against you?" "Well, not exactly," stuttered the patient, now starting to realize that the tide was rapidly turning against him. His allegation that I was obviously just a "typical" dental shyster out for the money without an honest diagnostic bone in my body really rankled the judge. "Dr. Mayputz did not cause your periodontal disease, which is well documented in your radiographic and written records, nor did he dentally treat you. And he properly suggested for you to see a periodontist," the judge angrily stated and then sarcastically asked, "You have no case, so why are you here?" Mr. Pisspotte began to rattle off a few manufactured grievances against the dental profession in general before the judge stopped him in midsentence and pronounced, "Case dismissed, and I never want to see you badmouthing dentistry in my courtroom again!" I glanced at the judge and threw my arms up in an apologetic gesture, in essence that he had to go through another farce with me again. He grinned and mouthed "I'm sorry" to me and then we all dispersed. Nothing was mentioned about the patient still owing me money, however. That would be a small-claims court case, and I was not going to pursue it. My appointed lawyer, who had not said a word during the entire ridiculous debacle, clapped me on the back in congratulations, got into his late model Beemer, and sped off. I had no afternoon patients scheduled that day as my dental assistant and I walked back to the office. With coffee mugs in hand, we sat down in my private room and relived the last two lawsuits against me. There was no laughter, just painful and stilted reminiscences while sipping hot liquid. Finally, I changed the subject slightly. "An old salt once told me in dental school that if a dentist could just get rid of that problematic twenty percent of total patients, she/he would be all set," I enunciated with a smirk on my face. "More like eighty percent with our scurvy lot," my assistant responded with an even bigger smirk on her puss. And she was probably right, you know. Of course if all dentists "cleaned house," the national drinking, divorce and suicide rates would plummet and we can't be skewing statistics, now can we?

31

"It Didn't Hurt Until You Touched It!"

Q.T. Torte was an immaculately dressed, youngish lawyer whose wife had the chintzy GHI dental insurance plan. The office I now worked at as an employee dentist took it as full payment for most dental procedures rendered. To make a profit from a plan like that you either had to be fast when treating a lot of likewise insured patients or pad the bill with work that was never done. Well, our office did not commit fraud but woe to the other dentists in our large group practice who were sluggishly slow; I'm not sure how they made money. Luckily, we accepted a plethora of other dental insurances which reimbursed us much better than GHI did. Anyway, Mr. Torte was in my schedule for a simple, single, one surface filling on an upper right first molar. His preliminary screening by my dental assistant T.A. attested to the fact that he was in no discomfort and that the tiny carious lesion had been noted during his previous hygiene appointment. Furthermore, his x-rays were within normal limits with nothing exciting to look at. He was dentally and medically boring except for that niggling cavity in his tooth, one that he was not even aware of. T.A. always briefed me about each patient and the treatment to be accomplished, and I scoffed at the simplicity of such a niggardly filling. I jokingly stated that perhaps she could do it and let me have some more time to check my email messages or Facebook posts. We both chuckled at that thought as we entered the operatory and anticipated a quick resolution to his dental problem. I gave him a shot of 3% Carbocaine, a short acting local anesthetic, scanned the x-ray of the tooth as a cursory gesture and after a few minutes began, and then finished. It was easy-peasy. It took me a total of five minutes tops of working time, and he didn't feel a darn thing. He was impressed and thankful as he shook my hand in delight. I just smiled a cocky grin as my dental assistant dismissed him. It was all routine and all went well, but did it? No, it did not. I didn't make much money on him or not at all because of the poor reimbursement from GHI; however, that was not the pressing issue. The problem was why was he back in my schedule with a raging toothache a week after I had more than successfully filled his cavity? Before I entered the dental treatment room, my assistant had wisely snapped a new digital x-ray of the offending tooth to see what the hell was going on. I looked at the radiographic image on the computer in my private office and did not see anything amiss; nothing that would indicate the level of discomfort that he was experiencing. The filling looked perfect and there was no abscess above the roots; the tooth looked fine. Perhaps the bite was off; sometimes that could bring on painful episodes until it was relieved. I anticipated administering some palliative therapy to Mr. Torte as I strode into the alcove of our previous jovial encounter. All the past good vibes in that room had evaporated as Mr. Torte glared at me and wanted satisfaction for a throbbing toothache that was escalating in severity. "It didn't hurt until you touched it!" he cried out in anger. And there it was, the punch in the gut, the proverbial saying that all dentists must contend with at least a few thousand times in their careers. Oh, boy. But it was true; his tooth did indeed hurt even when I tapped on it ever so gently. I proceeded to check his bite, which was perfect, and then applied a special desensitizing solution, all in the hopes of topically sedating it. It did not work. Nevertheless, I saw no cause as to why it should be behaving so badly. When I tried to explain to the patient that oftentimes it takes a few days to weeks for a tooth to calm down after a composite restoration is placed, he did not buy it and accused me of butchering the job. My assistant T.A. assured him that he was in capable hands, all to no avail. "So, why is it killing me if he's so good?" he spit out at her. Finally, I gave him a very small dose of a local anesthetic and that seemed to alleviate his immediate distress, at least for a few moments so that my dental assistant and I could collect our thoughts as to what should come next. Thinking privately, I knew from experience that once in a blue moon a highly placed nerve inside a tooth could become so traumatized, even during a routine procedure, that it could become nonvital and infected. This would cause intractable pain usually necessitating a root canal to save the tooth. And there was that dreaded word: Root Canal! Lawyer or not, I pulled up my britches and told him the possible treatment sequelae for a toothache that would not go away, namely a root canal or extraction. So, what had started as a fun-filled, tooth-filling event had instead morphed into a possible lawsuit due to my supposed dental incompetence. Fortunately, he worked for the State and was not in a private law firm. But I'm sure he had friends in the litigation world. I had exhausted my exculpatory spiel to him and sort of persuaded him that things like this sometimes happen and that I was truly sorry. And I was. Hopefully there would not be a court summons in my mailbox any time soon. My assistant and I made a referral for him to a local endodontist as Mr. Torte seemed resigned to his dental fate, until he blew up once more upon finding out that the root canal specialist did not participate with his shitty GHI plan. He would have to pony up big bucks for "my error," as he bluntly put it. Now he was really mad. I could tell that my assistant wanted to scream out loud that it was not our fault that he had such lousy dental insurance But I cut her off just as she defensively tried to utter that statement. Things were going from bad to worse in a hurry. There were three intelligent human beings in a room yet all positive communication had ceased, all because of a molar that was probably internally, anatomically, fucked up. It just wasn't fair. Finally, Mr. Torte saw the futility of further arguing and realized that I could not "fix" things. He got up and abruptly stalked out of the office, clutching that specialist referral form in his chubby left hand. And we never heard from him or his wife again, but I did find that important piece of paper we had given him in the office parking lot days later, rain soaked and battered. I'm not sure how he had his severe toothache resolved. And I never received a subpoena for a deposition either. Thank goodness. The unfortunate take-away from this story is this: Most patients will turn on you in a second. And in today's hyper-victimized, entitled and stressed-out world, it is happening more and more frequently.

32

Sugar Daddy Dentistry

The appointment schedule on the operatory computer screen read that a Mrs. Berserkowitz was coming in at eleven o'clock for a prosthodontic consultation. The small note under her name said that she had multiple dental implants placed by an oral surgeon in Connecticut but now lived close by. It seemed like a routine type of consult for me as my dental assistant T.A. and I talked a little shop and a little nonsense in my private office just before she arrived. After she was seated in the dental chair my dental assistant came to collect me but not before informing me about the patient's medical history and showing me her out-of-state x-rays. So far, so good. Now, whether out of stupid stereotypical ignorance or personal experience, I fully expected to encounter a stately Jewish woman of means as I sauntered down the hallway heading toward the treatment room. I entered the operatory and was shocked to see a beautiful, very well-endowed, sexily attired young woman with luxurious, jet black hair reclined rather provocatively in the dental chair. She was café-au-lait complected and of an obvious Far Eastern ethnicity. I doubted that she was of Japanese or Chinese heritage

because the assets on her upper torso were huge. But
maybe they were fake? And what was that racially similar
looking adolescent boy doing in the room as well? I recall
just standing there at first, altering my puzzled gaze
between the hottie, the teenager and my assistant, and
waiting for someone to start talking. I sat down and in
broken English the young man filled me in. He and his
mom had moved to this country after her recent nuptials
in Thailand, their native nation. Then he briefly explained
her earlier dental treatment as best as he could. What a kid.
He had willfully decided to miss study hall, lunch and gym
at his middle school to dutifully come in and help out his
mom as an interpreter because although smiling alluringly
at me, she did not speak a lick of English. But perhaps she
understood more than she let on? And the last name was
indubitably her new husband's. And though slightly
curious, I did not know if the young lad had come with
the bride as a package deal or was a product of the
marriage to Mr. Berserkowitz. The teen Thai appeared to
be about twelve years old, so probably not the latter.
Nevertheless, now we were all on the same page and I
could begin my dental examination. Mrs. Berserkowtz's
dentition had been expertly restored with a bevy of fine
crowns and bridges throughout her mouth. The only places
needing additional therapy were the remaining bilateral

spaces in her lower jaw. The dental implants had already been placed and my job was to affix crowns on them, as per the normal continuum of the prosthetic process. However, I did notice a slight hiccup. The radiographs of her teeth seemed to show a stark lack of bone around the implanted fixtures in her jawbone. Now, it was possible that the surrounding bone had deteriorated since the implants were placed or, alternatively that it was the best outcome of a dicey dental situation, with the oral surgeon giving her a guarded prognosis at best. Since I could not easily refer her back to Connecticut, I decided to phone the oral surgeon in question after she departed and get the scoop on the situation. With our mutual introduction and exam concluded Mrs. Berserkowitz and her son left the office, but not before scheduling a lengthy future visit for actual treatment. And I marveled at the notions that neither the proposed work nor the money required seemed to faze her in the least. I was glad of that; here was a patient that I didn't have to coerce, cajole or haggle with in order to get a good dental outcome. I ended up calling her distant oral surgeon and he assured me all was *Kosher* with her four dental implants, and to restore them with confidence. I noted that fact in her computer chart and ordered the necessary parts and pieces for the upcoming building bonanza. The appointment day arrived and as I calmly walked into the operatory I immediately noticed two things: Firstly, a Sugar Daddy candy that was bizarrely lying in plain sight on the countertop behind the patient's head and, secondly, a portly, balding, White dude slumped against the far wall in the room. While internally chuckling and rolling my eyes, I quickly secreted the caramel sweet into a drawer and then noticed my dental assistant giggling. SHE had brought it in as a joke and it worked; however, hopefully no one saw it but me. The older gentleman spoke up in perfect English and told me that he was her husband and would be accompanying her at all times as a translator and comforter. His adopted son could no longer take any more time off from school. He also matter-of-factly mentioned that nothing was too good for his wife and then asked if I noticed her many physical attributes, which he had paid for. Really? As if I didn't see that coming! However, I did not reply to his lascivious and leading questions and decided to be utmost professional in dealing with this couple. Mentally I remembered some years prior that a non-descript, middle-aged, misogynistic White male patient had regaled me with tales of his sexual exploits with young and purportedly willing women in Thailand. He said it was worth it to jet clear across the globe during his vacations and be treated like royalty upon landing. He further added, "If you have the bills, you can get some thrills." Supposedly, he was constantly and fervently surrounded by doting women during his inexpensive times there and felt like a king. I recall slightly recoiling while listening to him brag and intuitively deduced that those glamorous, under-aged hookers purposely masqueraded themselves as worthy courtesans while simultaneously leading lives of poverty and desperation. Anyway, Mrs. Berserkowitz may have been one of those street tarts and started out at the low end of life but married into great wealth that seemingly had no limits. Perhaps she was one of the lucky ones who was able to enrapture and capture Moby's Dick, and the great white whale that went with it. Anyhow, as I began the restorative process, I noticed that her gums around the implant healing sites did not appear healthy at all. Everything had dramatically changed for the worse within a two-week period and I was stunned. I reviewed the x-rays once more and remembered that her oral surgeon had given me the green light to proceed with my end of the treatment. But things suddenly looked bad. I had treated thousands of such cases and knew healthy oral tissues when I saw them. Something was amiss and I gently tried to tell her, through Mr. Berserkowitz, of course. The patient started to weep yet her husband didn't panic or look distressed in any way. He just took it in stride as if setbacks with his young bride were commonplace and to be expected. He acted more like her father than husband, if you know what I mean. Cool, calm and collected, he asked me about the options, and we had a reasonable conversation. I suggested she see her oral surgeon at once because I feared the implants were not thriving. And that meant postponing the prosthetic phase of treatment indefinitely until that fluky implant condition could be ameliorated. Fast forward four months and she was ready for a second attempt with me. Mr. Berserkowitz stated that the oral surgeon was as baffled as me and ended up replacing two of the implants and surgerizing the other ones. All four were now out of the bullpen and ready to be crowned. And then I did my thing! Fast forward a few weeks and there sat Mrs. Berserkowitz in my chair for a recall visit, grinning from ear to ear and complimenting me in Thai about her beautiful smile, or so said her banal husband. I checked the newly installed crowns and again noticed the gums around them starting to look soggy-boggy and spongy. Were the dental implants in jeopardy again, and this time all four at once? I had to tell Mr. Berserkowitz and he just sighed and grunted. "Those aren't the only implants that are failing," he blandly stated. "We are on the way shortly to her plastic surgeon's office," he further added. I felt bad that his hot wife seemed to be rejecting well-meaning and well paid for bodily accoutrements, including her bionic teeth. Granted most of her embellishments were for his titillation but, hey, I assumed she also derived some benefits from them. But there was a happy ending to this story. When I saw them again in a few months time, the midline of her busty cleavage seemed straight and the gingival health around her dental implants had greatly improved. None of the four crowns were mobile and new x-rays revealed a normal bony integration of said implants. I was amazed because spontaneous remissions of deleterious dental conditions are rare. Mrs. Berserkowitz was all smiles again and even her husband smirked a bit. Was it his money and patience that finally vanquished all those medical and dental demons that had bedeviled his Thai prize? Or maybe she started taking vitamins? I did not know. It's a marvelous mystery to this day.

33

Bridge Over Troubled Payment

I couldn't resist lifting most of that title from Simon and
Garfunkel's seminal hit ballad of 1970 because it is apropos
for this next vignette. Mr. A. Skippaar had repeatedly
warned me about his upcoming divorce and imminent
resettlement in another state yet I repeatedly chose to
ignore his words. Like the boy who cried wolf, the rest of
the office staff had also heard his domestic tale of woe for
years and never paid it too much mind either. So now it
was finally time to restore his missing front teeth with a
long-span, permanent porcelain bridge, which he insisted
on doing quickly because he was leaving very soon. Well,
we all knew that simply wasn't true and I basically
humored his personal saga. His crappy CSEA dental
insurance was through his wife and he would be
responsible for half of the bridge fee based on our contract
with the insurance carrier. X-rays and documents were
submitted to CSEA but instead of waiting to get its final
approval, as was the office norm, we decided to begin
treatment in anticipation of a positive nod from it. I mean,
he seemed to be in a God-awful hurry, so I acquiesced to
his demands. He wasn't a bad guy, a bit blustery and

insistent of character, but what did you expect from a longtime salesman? So we began and finished. And it turned out to be a gorgeous piece of pottery that blended in perfectly with his existing dentition. The shade and shapes of the artificial ivories were right on the money. The top of the line, indestructible, zirconium-infused ceramic prosthesis was probably the finest dental work I had ever accomplished in my long and storied career thus far. Well, at least long, that is. Anyway, I absolutely loved the outcome as did the patient. Other staff members paraded into and out of my operatory just to get a glimpse of the "magnificent bridge" that was shining in his pie hole. I was smiling, my dental assistant T.A. was smiling, and the patient was congratulated by all comers as he kept on grinning. And then Mr. Skippaar skipped town and skipped out on paying anything. But he did text us a forwarding address and phone number. Wait just a minute. You mean he had been serious about leaving all along? What about the paltry greenbacks he and CSEA owed us? He had promised to pay the balance once the insurance company had paid its portion. However, now the befuddled staff informed me that a letter they received from CSEA read that his spouse had previously divorced him from her policy, and it would pay us *bupkis*! An angry staff member somehow contacted him at his new address via a landline telephone and he jovially stated that he would be glad to pay the balance once the insurance company paid up. And if CSEA did not fork over the sawbucks neither would he. And then he rudely slammed down the phone at his end which shocked my surprised receptionist. When we called the supposedly soon-to-be ex-wife, she laughed long and hard and applauded him for pulling a good swindle. She told us that he knew all along that he was no longer covered by her insurance and had no intention of parting with any of his money. She then berated the receptionist and told her to fuck off and never call again. She wasn't our patient and probably enjoyed telling us off like that. When we valiantly contacted CSEA, a senior insurance manager informed us that the patient's coverage had recently been terminated and it owed us nothing. A big, fat ZERO! Of course, we could have pursued Mr. Skippaar though legal channels but dealing with collections in Alaska would be tricky. That was a dead end. And I suppose we could have insisted on speaking to the highest echelon of mediocre minions and mental midgets employed by CSEA insurance to plead our case but ultimately did not. I already knew the formulaic answer that we would receive in response. In any event it had been a sorrowful and expensive ending to a brilliant dental performance on my part. As an employee dentist, I ended up not receiving my share of the loot, nor did the office. And on top of that, who had to pay the dental laboratory for that expensive bridge? That's right, yours truly. I had been a duped stupe, actually losing cash on the whole goddamn deal. If I had been the owner of the practice, I could have written it off as bad debt but as a flunky lackey, I had to take it on the chin and in the pocketbook. And I can't say live and learn because after nearly thirty years in the "business" I should have "learned" by now. I hope his bridge collapses someday but more than likely it will not!

34

The Bad Penny

Every dental practice has at least one or two, or a shitload. You know, the patient that you just can't finish and get rid of, the one that seemingly has a black cloud following her/him around. The one whose treatment keeps faltering and blowing up; you fix one thing, two more break. The one in whom you valiantly adjust, trim, repair, modify, and replace, and then lose your financial shirt over. That kind of patient; the bad penny that keeps on showing up! But how could I have known that an initially trivial dental procedure would have me pulling out all the stops and any of my remaining hair, all to no avail as I vainly flailed away in failure. And things started out so good, too! It was an "easy" case, and the patient was so glad to have met me. She badmouthed her previous female dentist up the wazoo and worshipped my initial forays into her allegedly mishandled mouth. I could stop this ditty now – you readers already know the outcome….However, here are a few more words for your prurient entertainment. Initially, she presented to my office with a faulty and poorly made crown that kept coming off. She had a legitimate gripe about the continuing saga of having it glued back on in shorter and shorter intervals by a dentist she began to revile. I logically decided to remake it much to her delight and common sense. Oh, boy, we both were on the same page and on the way to success. But wait, good fortune was not about to smile upon us that quickly, if ever. Unbeknownst to me, she was an occlusal nomad (she never bit the same way twice – a very rare condition), had a rapidly failing dentition that I ultimately could not save, and personality-wise was a bit of a bitter butt-nut. The new molar crown was seated to fit the existing lower partial denture and cemented with permanent resin cement. Goody, goody gumdrops I was done, and the office only needed to collect the dental insurance payment and her portion of the copay. Ha, ha. Three practices and twenty-eight frustrating years later, now with top and bottom implant-supported dentures, she was still showing up like clockwork in my schedule. It got to the point where I would glance at the operatory computer screen and start having a panic attack due to seeing her blasted name there. I would complain to the front desk ladies that a half-hour appointment was just not long enough for her. And it never was! There were always more things to accomplish and "correct" than I had time for. On top of that she sarcastically complained during the entire allotted session as my dental assistant T.A. scowled, watching me frantically try to think outside the box and perform prosthodontic magic that was not described in any known dental textbook. To make matters worse I had remade her extensive artificial dentition from scratch many times over at no charge out of a sense of loyalty, guilt and empathy. And that only added to my incessant stress and monetary misery whenever I treated her. Even my dental laboratory stopped charging me after a while out of a sense of sympathy. Luckily, as an employee dentist, I retired from the practice and retired from treating her, too. Thank goodness. But it wasn't completely her fault or mine, as I retroactively examined my ulcer-inducing tenure with her. It must have been an act of a vengeful dental god, at least that's the story I am sticking to. But as I continue to work once more at a distant dental office as a part-time employee prosthodontist, I cannot help but think of who she is needlessly needling now. Hopefully, the hapless new sap, I mean dentist, can take it and can take better care of her than I did. Let's hope that someday soon there is an ending for her, a dental ending that is.

35

Defensive Driving

The phrases "do no harm" and "it's a litigious society out there" effectively put the brakes on my initial hubris as a young dentist. I don't remember from whence I heard them, but those short sentences have managed to keep my dental fervor in check all these years. However, is it really to my patients' or my benefit to continually practice judiciously, meticulously and conservatively? Possibly. Is practicing by the K.I.S.S. (Keep It Simple Stupid) principle the best route to go? Probably, at least for a gun-shy, grey-muzzled, and formerly cocky prosthodontist like me. And although my dental fears may be unjustified, they seem to have only gotten worse over the long decades of practice. Please, allow me: Like a barely alive warrior scarred after many battles, although only mentally, most dentists get less brave as time marches on. I am one of those. Patients sometime ask me how long I have been a dentist. I usually sarcastically reply that dental years are "officially" measured in dog years. Just multiply my years of service by seven. Two hundred forty-five years seems about right, and, boy is this basset hound old and tired! Born "hardwired" hypervigilant and overly inquisitive, my character flaws were validated early on by that seminal, mid-sixties, television public service catchphrase to help thwart car accidents: "Watch out for the other guy." As a child I'd sit back and relax while watching Davey and Goliath shorts on the boob tube Saturday mornings and then tense up whenever those well-meaning traffic-related slogans would pierce my eardrums. I recall those words to this day and continually drive AND practice dentistry "defensively" whenever possible. In addition to that bygone blip that seemed to resonate with me, my mild paranoia and observant nature proved to be an advantage as I maneuvered through life. I was an excellent dental student years later due in large part because of watching out for any untoward abnormalities in patients' mouths, and intuitively asking the right questions about their oral health. But enough about me. Nah, just kidding! Anyway, as I have gained more experience and insight while becoming a cranky, crotchety and cynical prosthodontist, my "defensive" dental skills have also greatly improved. Gone is the brash and handsome (well, at least brash) do-gooder full of piss and vinegar who could conquer caries with a single stroke of the dental drill. Instead, what's left is a dentist who has pretty much seen and heard it all. That kind of attitude is undoubtedly a defense mechanism from years of getting my rhubarb rubbed the wrong way.

All those anxious, button-pushing patients and their mental-dental gymnastics that I formerly and willingly accepted have reduced me to practicing a form of no nonsense, non-heroic and stoic style of dentistry. When a female or male patient seems to "fall in love" with me, I just roll my eyes and quickly disentangle myself from that minefield in a hurry. Nothing leads to trouble faster than the flirtatious expectation of dental excellence that unexpectedly turns out sideways. The scorn of the woman attached to that unruly molar can cause much heartache and distress for the hapless doctor who should have seen it coming. A dentist can go from a lover to goat (and NOT greatest of all time) in a barnyard second. When an Oshkosh-clad male patient angrily wants me to hurry up and finish all his neglected dental work in one session because of an upcoming hillbilly hoedown in the Ozarks, the first thing I do is recommend another dentist. No more dental bullying, no more bullshit allowed! I can only do what I can do, in the time period allotted, period! I've become more like a lowly amoeba or paramecium that recoils from noxious stimuli. Even my dental language has changed over time. My younger and vigorous version would confidently predict outcomes with ease and then sweat profusely to get them accomplished, oftentimes getting underpaid and overworked in the process. Not so much anymore. Now I routinely and frequently use carefully chosen words and phrases such as maybe, we'll see how it goes, sometimes it may work out, here's to hoping, start praying, are you feeling lucky, etc. Conservative, well-thought out dentistry without a hard sell or phony optimism is what I preach and practice with the dental onus placed squarely on the patient. Personal responsibility and cooperation are a two-way street and I make patients aware of that fact. In addition, what about all those difficult to diagnose situations? You know, when the dentist stares at the "normal" x-ray and then at the "normal" tooth in question only to be sniped at by the patient who insists that he/she is in excruciating pain? I have been in that unenviable position thousands of times. Sometimes you just don't know what to do. Do you tell the patient to take Advil and to suck it up and wait a few more weeks? Do you paint some fluoride and desensitizing varnish on that offensive premolar, or do you jump right in and start a root canal procedure? Some dentists would absolutely do the latter. By contrast, I would rather lose a patient than do something premature and possibly harmful in the long run. But that's me. Sure, I now say "I don't know" with ease and may have turned into a cuspid-coward after suffering from all the dental carnage over the decades, but the often-simplified solutions I offer are prosthodontically sound, WELL-DOCUMENTED, and hopefully long lasting. I also find it better to lowball a dental treatment and then have the patient celebrate with a "victory" highball when things turn out better than expected. However, I may be unique in my dotage for I still hear stories about aggressive, seasoned, dental hammers out there nailing everything in sight, including a lot more than their wives.

36

The Blame Game

The moment of truth has arrived. The standing "Brady Bunch" in the cramped operatory is plastered against the far wall, holding its collective coats, hats and breath. And Grandpa "Brady" is in the chair, anxiously awaiting the insertion of his new dentures, the ones which took three months to make, the ones which passed each step with flying colors as to the shade of teeth, proper bite and fit. Grandpa is excited as my dental assistant chirps incessantly while obnoxiously describing me in glowing terms, over and over again. Then I walked in and unceremoniously studied the finished plates and slightly adjusted them as needed prior to prying them into Grandpa's tight oral orifice. This was it; they would either have suction and a perfect occlusion or be pieces of shit. They were pieces of shit, with the top one embarrassingly falling down upon placement. Although looking alright in my gloved hands, they did not stay in place in his mouth as required. The bottom prosthesis just laid there but the upper one should have adhered snugly to the upper ridge and stayed put all by itself. Of course, sometimes it takes a few days for the gums to conform to a new denture, but my decades of experience told me otherwise. It was wiser to start over rather than *putz* around and "make" it fit. However, first I had to give a satisfactory answer to the puzzled peanut gallery whose bewildered communal stare went right through me. My dental assistant had mysteriously disappeared as usual leaving me quite alone to face the firing squad. It was not a pleasant task to inform the homely, *home crowd* that Grandpa would not be getting his teeth that day and that a new upper had to be manufactured. I mean I could have slapped some denture adhesive into it or relined it with a temporary material and bullshitted my way out of trouble, but my prosthodontic pride and the money spent was at stake. Nevertheless, this event had occurred to me numerous times over my career. Although there could be mitigating oral anatomic factors negating a good outcome, oftentimes there were no good explanations for a poor result. On top of that, all the textbook dental rules had been followed precisely; after all, this was my specialty. And crap like this still happened. As a certain former president would have whined, "it was so unfair;" but it was in fact a normal part of my abnormal dental life. However, I did not panic or stammer; I just matter-of-factly blamed the dental laboratory that had made them. That's right, when in doubt, blame the lab. To admit failure is to have the patient lose confidence in the dentist and that just ain't happenin.' The frowning crowd dispersed as I began the process of taking new impressions to make a new upper denture for Grandpa. The lower one was deemed satisfactory and could remain. I can tell you that everything turned out swell the second time around with relieved smiles from the relatives and especially Grandpa, who left grinning and satisfied. But I was not kidding about blaming dental laboratories. Because they are an integral and intimate part of virtually every restorative dental practice, they are an absolute necessity in dentistry. But at the same time they are seldom seen or heard outside of dentistry circles, quietly fabricating crowns, bridges, partials, and complete dentures, etc. Few patients even know they exist or what they do for dentists. That's why they are an easy target of dentists' derisions. How does a patient know if the dentist or the lab fucked up? It's the dentist's word against a mysterious "lab" somewhere in California, one that "purposely" messed up the crown so that it won't seat properly, or got the shade wrong because the supposedly "certified" foreign-born lab technicians that work there are so stupidly negligent. Gee whiz, dental laboratories, or is it lavatories, are real pieces of work, aren't they? Not really. Sometimes the "problem" is due to a dentist's shoddy impressions or unrealistic demands which are placed upon the lab. The crappy work can flow both ways and there is never a winner, only a satisfied patient in the end. And secretly, most dentists are proud of the distinct labs they use and rely on them heavily for virtually all the products that get inserted and cemented into patients' oral cavities. Specially trained technicians are the ones responsible for the gorgeous aesthetic veneers and crowns that we dentists take credit for. Loyalty from both ends is a factor as well, for if something is amiss or goes awry, it usually gets remade at no cost to the dentist. In other words, if the dentist is not happy, neither is the lab because both parties wish to get paid and maintain a professional relationship. It is wise to select a lab that fits a certain budget and dental style, however. Oftentimes a dentist has to shop around for awhile before finding that certain synergistic and mutually profitable partnership. I have been with my select dental laboratories for many years and have no intention of jumping ship although I am not above belittling them in front of patients, especially when it comes to saving my fragile ego and reputation. It's an easy way out when things don't fit or fall apart, or just plain look bad. Thusly, we dentists tell a few white lies now and again and pretend to take our wrath out on "those laboratory idiots" but in the end usually do the procedure over together with them, hopefully with a better outcome the next time around!

37

Continuing Education?

What a hot topic, and there's so much to say about it. Let's begin. Most states mandate a certain amount of non-online continuing education within a stated triennial period in order to maintain a dental license in good standing. Many dentists dutifully sign up for three or four courses (7 credit hours apiece) every January, pay three to four hundred dollars a pop for each lecture, and then cancel patients on those certain Fridays when they will be gone from the office to "larn about dem toofers." My beef with this system is this: If the state education department (the body that licenses dentists) is so adamant about these learning protocols, why doesn't IT pay for them, and reimburse the dentists for the time off, as well? It's the edumacation department's idea, not mine. Why do I have to hand over MY valuable time and money for something that only MIGHT be good for me? And lately there have also been a plethora of additional and mandatory webinar classes to take for periodic recertification in substance abuse/opioid prescribing methods, CPR, infection control/hazcom compliance, HIPAA standards, etc. And to make matters worse, no one from the "Nanny State" bothers to send a reminder for these "extra" conferences but secretly audits licensee records to make sure dentists are in compliance and up to date. It's an intrusive gotcha game that dentists have unfortunately gotten used to, and there is nothing we can do about it. Anyway, I am used to sitting numbly on hard, metal folding chairs in the rear of large lecture halls while periodically getting educated, much like I did in pharmacy college and dental school. As a very long-haired but clean-shaven student, you would have reliably found me in the back row, against the wall, and as far away from the lectern as possible. It was my hippie-inspired, nose-thumbing style back then, but it did not prevent me from graduating summa cum laude and third in my dental school class. Anyhow, as I presently survey the crowd in front of me at these mandated group dental meetings, now with a balding and grey-haired pate, I see the same old college paradigm at work. The same, lame, suck-up, lap dogs sitting at the altar, lapping up the drivel dribbling out of the lecturer's cake hole while diligently taking copious notes. Nothing has changed. Most of those attentive attendees are women; however, there are some dubious menfolk among them as well. And the non-stop, softball questions lobbed up from that pious crowd are typically useless for the rest of us. It seems as though there is this personal fawning going on between the front row and the speaker. What are they buttering him/her up for? There is no need. There are no brownie points awarded this time around for being a winsome, goody-two-shoes pupil. We should be cynical and callous adults by now, well, at least one dentist is. However, old habits are hard to break and I silently laugh at the "misguided classroom cretins" whenever I attend these symposiums, in much the same manner as I did years ago as a taciturn and savvy student. Some things remain the same! But wait, things weren't always like this. Why did I turn out to be so jaded and anti-establishment? I don't know. I had forgotten that as a once young dentist, I also had been a featured local speaker numerous times at these dental soirees, with my own Kodak slides, Kodak slide projector and portable Polaroid screen. (This was way before slick power point presentations via computer). I tried my hardest to portray an image of knowledge and brilliance as a prosthodontic specialist, but the real reason was to solicit referrals for my budding practice by showcasing a bunch of good-looking patient smiles in a darkened room. Unfortunately, the referrals never materialized, and I retreated to the back row, literally and figuratively. Perhaps it was my lack of public speaking skills or maybe the insane jealousy that emanated from area wannabe prosthodontists that put a damper on my nascent lecture circuit? It was most likely the latter, I surmised. There were turf wars going on back then. Many offices were like black holes or Black Flag Roach Motels where "Roaches check in, but they don't check out." A patient entered but never left. Referral to a specialist? Yeah, right! I was still busy enough in my office, just not doing the quantity of reconstructive dentistry I thought I should be. I recall feeling chastened and chagrined and wondered if there was some magic I had lacked as an orator and signed up for an expensive two-day denture course in Delaware presented by a "famous" elderly prosthodontist whose articles of wisdom regularly appeared in national dental journals. I would get triple the continuing education credits, visit the "Hypocrite State," where our current POTUS hails from, and possibly pick up some pointers on how to be a more efficacious and dynamic teacher; in case I decided to play that game again. The car trip was long but uneventful, as was the lodging at the swanky Embassy Suites Hotel in the small city. The event was paid for by we signed-up *schlubs* and cosponsored by a local dental lab, ballyhooed as the best in town. It was supposed to be a production extravaganza complete with finger foods to nosh on and refreshing liquids to quaff them down with and I fully expected a standing-room-only crowd to hear the famed doctor reveal his dental "secrets." Arriving a bit early at the venue, I anxiously glanced around and saw dentists trickling into the vacuous room to take padded seats behind me and at that moment recalled the immortal words of Flounder from the movie *Animal House*: "Oh, boy, is this great?" I was all atwitter and ready to listen and learn from the best! Even I had a notebook and pen at the ready and became my own worst nerdy nightmare as I took a seat at the front of the oversized auditorium and waited for the *Maestro* to enter. The slide projector was percolating, burly male hotel assistants were singly positioned in the distant four corners, and all that was lacking was a light spectacle and some WWE-type raucous intro music to announce the main combatant, Dr. J.T. But wait, was that the whole crowd: Nineteen woebegone females and one handsome male, besides myself? (I re-counted the attendees a few times just to be sure). That spacious place could have held a legitimate Royal Rumble wrestling match or an evangelical Christian Holy Roller service and yet only a sprinkling of dentists showed up for the Main Event. How disappointing and ignominious. Dr. J.T. entered and started right in, before we could even click our pens into useful writing implements. Charismatic, stately, and slightly portly, Dr. J.T. first dispensed with seemingly inappropriate personal stuff, such as showcasing slide after slide of his seven scantily clad and beautiful former wives, dozens of offspring and of his current, young sexy flame. He was in his late sixties and she was in her late twenties, at most. He told us matter-of-factly that in his backwoods, "hillbilly hamlet" in West Virginia, he was considered the best catch in town and women of all ages were lined up to be the next Mrs. J.T. I instantly wheeled around and fully expected a boycott, walkout or at least loud grumbling from the femme contingent but instead was utterly surprised at seeing all the blushing and longing faces. What was going on here? Were those lady dentists really into his patriarchal, misogynistic and anti-feminist act? It was as if they had willingly signed up for this course while knowing about his politically incorrect and sexist rhetoric ahead of time. Was that it? Did they know him? Were some of them his ex-wives? No, that couldn't be it; they were all Plain Janes! I was puzzled as he at last launched into his lecture. It was the usual fanfare of perfect outcomes on perfect and well-satisfied patients, male and female. Gag me. And, of course, he mentioned the obscene fee he charged for dentures and how the financially bankrupt and derelict lowlifes in his area eagerly ponied up the greenbacks necessary to have false teeth made by him. Was he a god, or at least a demigod like Hercules? At that point I hunkered down like a box turtle and let his ensuing arrogant words glance off my "shell" without riling my inner sarcastic demon. I desperately wanted to speak out numerous times and perhaps call out that bragging blowhard but kept my beak shut and effectively clammed up. After all, I had paid a good dollar for this bodacious bonanza and wisely decided to silently stick it out, unlike my neck! Oh, there were a few pearls thrown out here and there which I thought might be useful in my practice; however, the majority of his spiel was a self-aggrandizing affair. Was that what I should do if I was ever invited to speak again? Mention a few salient dental points but mostly brag about myself and then reveal photos of my bikini-clad wife, Hottie Blondie? And then further talk about how lucky she was to be married to me? Ha, ha. I don't think so: not to the cynical and envious upstate New York dentists! They would eat me for lunch. Anyway, at the scheduled luncheon I overheard the women dentists tittering amongst themselves while we were in the short buffet line. It seemed as if most of them knew each other from previous encounters. And I had mistakenly thought they were from disparate parts of the country. Hmmm.... I boldly approached one of them, introduced myself and asked what the hell was going on. She was overly friendly and pointed out that she and her small cohort of female dentists were from differing parts of the nation and adoringly followed Dr. J.T. on his disjointed speaking tour. Were they "cult members" tailing a noted and dynamic impresario/buffoon and worshipping a man resembling that money-making fraud Tony Robbins? I was confused. And when I asked her if she and her friends also charged $6,000.00 per set of dentures, she demurely said no. "We don't pay the one thousand dollar tuition cost to learn how to soak patients or to be better prosthodontic dentists but to hobnob with "the Wizard" himself and to soak in his limelight," she added. How could they afford this kind of recurring and devotional tithing? What the eff? Were those ladies self-respecting dentists or starry-eyed band aids, groupies and backstage sluts? Was I at a Grateful Dead or Phish concert from yesteryear? I suddenly realized that they were paying for pricy presentations due to love and Dr. J.T. was in effect happily obliging and preaching to the choir. My head was spinning as I approached the other "man" in our midst and quickly realized he was of a similar disposition and ilk. He told me he idolized the doctor and someday hoped to be like him. Good lord, I needed to take a walk and I did. Was I and the few others present the only true outliers of the bunch? All those questions and no easy answers! I returned for the afternoon montage and took it in stride. Evening found me eating alone and sucking on a Wild Turkey double Manhattan in the hotel restaurant when who should stroll in but Dr. J.T. himself! And there was no entourage, no hangers-on with him, at least none that I could see. He recognized me from his talk and plopped down next to yours truly. Great, just great. As he gestured for a menu I steeled myself for more gratuitous and grandiose bullshit, but when he discovered that I was a fellow prosthodontist his mood drastically changed. For the next three hours we bonded as fellow specialists without any pretenses, anti-feminist jargon or condescension from either of us. Whether it was from the free-flowing libations and him letting down his hair I do not know, but his many revelations prompted me to recalibrate my attitude toward him. He was a *mensch* after all, and his stage routine was just a carefully choreographed cartoon. When I mentioned the harem of women and one man that fervently and reverently followed him around like sheep, he casually dismissed them as a paying posse of harmless hacks, and we both had a good laugh. "They pay me to be in my presence, so I love them back," he chortled as I winced a bit. When I mentioned his exorbitant office fees, he yelled that most of his bills were still unpaid, decades later. "It's one thing to charge but another to collect!" he spat out loud. It also turned out that most of his wealth came from being On the Stump and not from his dental practice receivables. "What about all the alimony you owe?" I drunkenly slurred. "All those dumb gals are good-looking but poor as shit. A curling iron, a bottle of

215

red nail polish, and Three Hots and a Cot are all they want; and I can still afford that," he slowly articulated with a twinkle in his good eye. We mutually parted company and I slowly side-winded to the nearest elevator. I went to bed with my head still buzzing from the booze and filled with Dr. J.T.'s revealing candor about the field of continuing dental education. It was eye-opening yet soporific. Maybe that last part was the bourbon talking. Anyhow, tomorrow was part two and I would be ready to absorb his last tidbits; ready and with a changed perspective about him and my fellow listeners. But would I ever give my own lectures again? Perhaps, but meanwhile I once again sit in the back row during continuing education snore fests and patiently doze while awaiting the all-important course codes to be announced at their completion. And during these sleep-inducing and restful junkets (with the emphasis on junk), I often silently reminisce about good-ole-boy Dr. J.T., his lineup of would-be paramours, and his loyal gaggle of followers. Ahh, those fucked up and fetid memories.

38

"Herodontics"

Although not an official dental word, I have seen and heard it enough to make it seem mainstream, at least in dentistry. What is it exactly? Well, simply put it is the act of heroically saving a patient's tooth or teeth, often by unorthodox means or with measures that have a low probability of success. The "grateful" patient usually saves some major bucks, is able to temporarily postpone the inevitable, and the challenged dentist is hailed a hero, at least for the day. An example would be a failing root canal: The patient can elect to extract the offending tooth and then treat the gap with a possible implant crown or fixed bridge; however, both are expensive propositions. Or the dentist could try to retreat the root canal in hopes of saving the tooth. If it works out, the patient just saved a boatload of money and the dentist walks on water for a short while. However, most of these "saving" attempts have a guarded prognosis and expiration dates associated with them. The scenarios are UNLIKE the 1972 FRAM oil filter commercials that succinctly stated: "The choice is yours; you can pay me now or pay me later." That saying implied that installing a relatively cheap oil filter obviated paying for a costly engine overhaul down the road. However, in dentistry coughing up a little dough now for a hurried fix is oftentimes NOT the correct choice for the choppers in question. They often come back to bite us at a future date and cost much more to repair! Alas, doing it right the first time can be problematic. The spoiled patient, once accustomed to "miracle cures," often seeks to continually coerce the dentist into being a Patch-O-Dontist or Bond-O-Dontist: one who will patch or bond the dental potholes only, and never do pricy and definitive dentistry. The "hero" dentist often becomes a patsy to the whims of many such patients and is in danger of relegating her/his practice to one of mediocrity and poverty. Do you repeatedly charge the patient for a filling that keeps falling out, one that never should have been placed? Probably not. Do you extract those periodically loose molars and plan for a partial denture, or do you give the patient an antibiotic prescription and hope for the best? Perhaps? In other words, the dentist who continually kicks the dental can down the road is not really "helping" the indigent and recalcitrant. She/he is merely enabling a dysfunctional dentition to barely keep functioning for the time being. At the same time the office reputation suffers and word spreads that the dentistry done there is subpar and the dentist, while a nice guy and purported savior, has no skills. Say, what? That's because the chemical axiom of "like attracts like" is in play here. A dentist who treats patients with subpar dentistry begets more patients wanting the same inferior treatments. Paradoxically, patients seeking comprehensive and detailed dentistry start avoiding the sloppy, chop-shop that practices "Herodontics." But I thought the dentist was truly helping people? Ha! And what about midcourse corrections. Let's say the bonded fillings used to raise the bite all came out and now the teeth in question need to be crowned? Who pays? The dentist, naturally; not the patient, who is used to a quick cure with no significant monetary depletion on her/his part. If the dentist insists, the patient will often fight back and threaten to leave the practice. And, worst of all, the dentist who abandons advanced dentistry gradually loses confidence and the skills he/she was taught in dental school. How do I know all of the above? Unfortunately, I've lived it, as have many dentists I have conversed with. I also have been guilty of acquiescing and doing the patient's bidding over and over again, especially as a young dentist eager to please a new and growing clientele. By the same token, and as a prosthodontist, I have seen many referral patients with more fillings than teeth whose dentists wanted me to crown a few. Those patients either refused to believe the old-timer or thought that he/she was incapable of doing fine dentistry. Either way they ended up in my specialist's chair and I did the requested and required dentistry. I felt bad for the referring dentists; I'm sure they could have easily done the work but did not. As an oldster myself now, I have a few caveats to add to my obviously snarky previous discourse. Firstly, as I have aged ungracefully, I have become dentally steeled and give my current patients only a few options for optimal dentistry that I know will last. It's nice to be empathetic but neither the patient nor I am being properly served with lousy dentistry. Secondly and lastly, there is one exception to the above sentences. I have practiced prosthodontics in big cities and in rural areas and let me tell you: small-town gossip can ruin you, whether you are a dentist or not. Sometimes I had to become a deft dental politician and to carefully evaluate the overall situation before I drilled away. Is it better to stay the battle for fear of reprisal from the patient and to keep the hard-earned goodwill around town, or does one dive in with an extensive and expensive treatment plan and potentially lose more than the patient? Those are tough decisions to make and practitioners wrestle with them daily. The "art of the compromise" is never easy but beware of being a dogmatically deluded dentist and only doing dilapidated dentistry; that kind of "hero" is at risk of becoming a broke buffoon.

39

Who's in Charge Here?

You would think that after three decades of stressful and grueling dentistry, I would have IT all figured out. Right? Wrong! And I'm talking about the music that is played in the dental office! During my initial salvo as a greenhorn associate dentist, working for a lying and despot dentist, I never gave much thought about the musical melodies emanating from the closed-off patient staging port. I recall that the front office reception area and the dental operatories were without tunes; only the waiting room had a constant but muted barrage of operatic music sidling out from speakers mounted in the ceiling. Knowing the pretentious and social-climbing owner as I did, it made perfect sense. Patients in the on-deck circle were most likely subliminally influenced into believing that their ensuing dentistry would be of the highest caliber and proficiency, mirroring legendary vocal virtuosos such as Mario Lanza, Enzo Stuarti and Enrico Caruso. I saw through the scheme but did not care at the time. I was too busy trying to make a dime. In my first practice as an owner, I loudly played what the "girls" in the office had listened to before I took over. It was a rinky-dink, top-40 station that played all the current hits. And the tunes were broadcast throughout the office, from the waiting area to the dental laboratory hovel in the back. I really did not listen; I was too busy pounding sand to really care one way or the other. I would occasionally look up out of the pigpen, pick out some familiar songs, but quickly got back to the slopping sweatshop again. The ladies in the office were happy, the patients did not complain and so I kept things as they were. After I moved slightly north to a swanky and suburban town, I began to pay attention to what I should play on the radio. Should I go opera, classic rock or something in-between? I had taken the same staff with me and "they" decided on going in-between, once more. The AM top hits were brayed throughout the practice and I did not really care. I was too busy to scrutinize the *tunage* while treating patients and trying hard to make money. After selling that practice and starting one from scratch in a city farther north, I decided to tone things down a bit with Nora Jones' CDs on my canned playlist offerings. She became the soothing and soulful songstress in my small and unique, boutique practice. I had one staff member, who doubled as my front office receptionist and dental assistant. I only practiced prosthodontics and surreptitiously wanted to deliver a patient experience of comfort and stress-free dentistry. And

I believe I achieved that while still managing to pay the bills. However, and with much reluctance and sadness, I sold that beloved office in 2011; all due to the federal government's bungled recession response in 2009. And I never owned another practice again. Then I became a free agent and a hired-gun dentist for anyone who wished my services. The offers came fast and furious and I decided to work in a large group practice doing my specialty only. It was OK, except for all the crappy general dentistry that emanated from that poorly run dental office. And the music was terrible, as well. Each room had a radio speaker which blasted out the top ten hits every five minutes. And you could not squelch that awful sound because there were no volume controls. Bruno Mars, Cher, Mumford and Sons, John Maier, etc., were singers and groups which were unwillingly foisted upon patients and me in an unfair and deleterious way, and on a daily basis to boot. I guess the dentist/owner liked that kind of shit, and it was shit! I quit that office after a two-year stint, and I think the music had something to do with it. My next employment was where I finally laid down the law. All this time I had been a hard rocker at heart, with artists like AC/DC, Ozzie Osbourne, Boston, Led Zeppelin, Judas Priest, Deep Purple, and The Cars being some of my favorite bands. I was once more employed in a large group setting yet had a positive say about the music played in the office on the days I was there. I loved the satellite offerings such as *Seventies at Seven* or *Classic Rock All Day*. Whenever my wedding song *Highway to Hell*, by AC/DC, came on the airwaves I had my dental assistant T.A. crank up the volume, much to the amusement of other staff members in the know. And whenever Foreigner played *Dirty White Boy* I would fondly reminisce about one of my former college nicknames with giggling female co-workers. But deep down I knew that the office personnel only tried to placate me on those certain days and did not really appreciate my taste in tunes. Whenever I entered the building there would be a mad dash to the receiver by specially appointed staff to quickly dial up an oldies rock station, lest I went ballistic. But I inadvertently caught the previous selections as I walked in and really did not mind, as long as they were squelched in a goddamn hurry! A majority of the ladies in the office enjoyed the hippity-hoppity (hip-hop) dance music. And besides listening to boffo fluff by pop tarts such as Brittany and Taylor, I heard they also juked and swayed to Five Cent, Ten Cent, Nellie, Lil Kim, Lil Wayne, Lil Nicky Z. and Cardi Gan Sweater. A minority even tried to sneak in channels playing lively fusions of jazz and funk; I called it junk! Nevertheless, country compositions were universally beloved and worshipped by ALL the female staff. This was

the great northeast, yet Minnie Pearl, Shania Twain and
Lyle Lovett had enormous influence over the rurally raised
"conservative girls" in this part of Upstate New York. I
mean, some of the office women hunted and fished, and
even wore camo to work when turkey hunting season was
upon us. It was no wonder that Buck Owens, Randy Travis
and Merle Haggard were the go-to artists who struck a
chord with those good-looking and God-fearing, redneck
babes. For the life of me I could not understand it, and for
a long while I put up with their stultified staff-room
grumblings about my radio preferences. But then we
reached a compromise. The end of the week would be
designated as "Country Fridays" and that went a long way
to keeping the peace in the office. However, I suffered
through endless karaoke-type sing-alongs in the hallways
during those bleak Fridays. The drunken wailing and
horse-references noisily excreting from the speakers were
oftentimes too much for me, but a deal was a deal.
Sometimes I took my musical frustrations out on my
dental assistant and mercilessly teased her about my faux
knowledge of Dolly Parton's or Tammy "Whiner"
Wynette's patented knee slappers. And don't get me started
about the times that those wealthy "country scoundrels"
Johnny Cash and Johnny Paycheck droned on in their
droopy voices. They often caused some of the female *staph*

to become emotionally "infected" as if the *gods* had finally spoken. I eventually quit practicing on those frightening Fridays but continued working on my "rock" days. Maybe it had been the aggravating sounds on that particular weekday that did me in and made me semi-retire? Perhaps. Finally, in my current part-time workplace, there is no communal music, period. The local AM and FM reception is very poor, and the owner is not interested in garnering expensive satellite service. However, each hygienist and assistant is allowed to play her favorite Pandora selections through the computer and the disparate dissonance is often breathtakingly ridiculous. I'm sure that Peruvian chants mixed with Scottish Sea Shanties and Gangsta Rap, alongside opera and Acid rock can be bewildering to the patients and their unaccustomed eardrums. Nevertheless, I am back in charge, at least for the few days a week that I am there, and only in my cramped dental operatory. But I'll take it. Long live rock-and-roll!

40

Same as it Ever Was

Like the recurring, haunting refrain from the 1980 Talking
Heads song *Once in a Lifetime*, those five titular words
continually taunt me, even in semi-retirement.
Unfortunately, regardless of technological advancements
and better techniques in dentistry, chairside etiquette and
mannerisms have not evolved to keep pace. It's still the
same old complaining, whining, sweating, and arm-chair
gripping belligerence of yesteryear, and yesterday for that
matter. And that sentiment applies to the patients as well!
It's the same as it ever was! Mrs. E. was a case in point.
Elegant, stylish and ever so polite, she had come in
specifically to have me fabricate complete dentures for her.
Mrs. E.'s chief complaint was that her current ones were
old and she wished them replaced with new ones, albeit
with bolder, brighter teeth to give her a winsome and
dazzling Hollywood smile; a no-brainer for a highly trained
prosthodontist like me. However, after more than three
numbing decades I can't believe I still fell for it. What am I
talking about? That malarkey of "sincere" pleading and
alleged cooperation from patients to rectify their dental
woes with a seemingly simple solution. Just change the

227

smile and that's all. Ha! Mrs. E. seemed genuine in wanting a "makeover" but somehow could not articulate it to me. And I could not get inside her head to learn all the nuances and intricacies of what she truly desired. She was looking for something but could not put her finger on it. We were not on the same page. I could only do the teeth. I could not change her face, her mental status or her outlook on life. These are the frustrating cases that drive dentists bonkers. Multiple different denture set-ups with various size teeth and shades were tried, all in vain. Visit after visit was filled with disappointing and disparaging remarks from her, as well. How could I not get things right the first time? Was I a prosthodontic specialist or not? She was just not happy. And when she eventually gave me the go-ahead to finish a set of false teeth, she came back to the office in tears because her nearly blind beagle did not recognize her. She clenched her fists in rage and wailed, "Why can't they be just like my old set?" To say I was exasperated would be a gross understatement. She further told me that perhaps she should turn into a beaver because that's what she looked like. Ouch! But didn't most movie stars have those big, bold and beautiful grins; the kind that she wanted? Oh well, I felt horrible nonetheless. But instead of multiple future agonizing appointments trying to guess at the oral appliances she had envisioned I cleverly fabricated a new

228

set of prostheses in wax only that precisely mimicked her old ones, even with the same color teeth. I sent her home with them to show her acquaintances, neighbors and any nearby varmints. As per my explicit instructions, and to prevent them from melting, I told her to carefully insert and then quickly remove them daily for a week's duration, and then come back to have them permanently finished in hard acrylic. She came back all right, but this time in a totally different mood. She was ecstatic and visibly beaming; she praised me up and down. And now her dog would recognize her as well! And she no longer lobbed any more rodent-resembling snide remarks in my direction, either. Glory be. So what were the takeaways from this story in addition to losing time, money and my remaining hair for the umpteenth time? Don't be a dentist? Don't treat difficult patients? Start drinking heavily, as Bluto (Blutarsky) advised Flounder to do in *Animal House*? Perhaps all three? Anyway, dentistry can be agonizingly difficult in the best of times but when you couple that with vague and unrealistic demands, it can be downright brutal. And Mrs. E. is a nice lady; and I'm sure she trumpeted my eventual success to family and friends. Accordingly, I had finally gotten IT right. Great, but at what cost to my sanity and stomach lining? Did she really think I was a heartless son of a bitch until I magically came through for her in the end? Are dentists considered good human beings only when things turn out right? What a disheartening profession I was in! But just as I started to think that I was sick and tired of continually getting emotionally snookered, I chanced upon an article stating that dentistry was the number one white collar profession to go into. Really? Who wrote that piece of happy and sappy drivel? And was it a narrative based on researched and viable facts; unlike OPINIONS derived from "anonymous" sources that are peddled as legitimate factoids by certain TV cable news networks? I thought back to my own dental school *daze* and the difference between then and now. Maybe something had changed? And it had. In my day female students were a voiceless minority and dental school was basically an old man's club which barely tolerated the fair sex within its chauvinistic walls. Nowadays, dental colleges across the country are overwhelmingly composed of matriarchally matriculated students. Wow! Are the femme enrollees pushing this unprecedented tome of positivity? And are the subsequently newly minted female dentists driving this "wonderful" portrayal of dentistry only to jump ship when the rigors of reality sink in? Could be. I personally know of many gals from my class of '86 who had the highest of grades and the brightest of futures yet quickly stepped off the toothy merry-go-round altogether after unsuccessfully trying to juggle sex, marriage, motherhood and that damn dental drill. Is that dynamic still happening? I don't know. I haven't read any current articles exploring that kind of hidden negativity and inconvenient truth. Anyway, and for whatever reasons, dentistry is the perceived "hot" job market to be in right now. Go figure. Anyhow, before I could continue exploring any feelings of burnout or ruminate on becoming an obsolete, part-time old-timer in the fourth quarter of my life and career, with no time-outs left, the Wuhan Flu descended on us. The politically lionized but ultimately disgraced and feckless governor of New York State hit the pandemic pause button and I became effectively jobless and in limbo as to working again. I suddenly found myself sequestered for months at home with my lovely wife, which wasn't a bad thing if you know what I mean. And guess what? I did NOT miss dentistry at all! Not at all. During that self-isolating lockdown, I realized that I had desperately needed this break, this forced sabbatical, all along. Who knew that the deadly viral plague would do me so much good? Who knew, indeed? During my involuntary repose, I exercised twice daily, ate well and cleared my head of the accumulated and nasty "dental-related clutter" that had been building up inside me for so long. It felt good to reset my priorities and be alive as a human being again.

But then, inevitably, most of us frontline dentists sadly picked up our feet and sullenly trundled back to work, while the killer novel virus was still raging and picking up steam. However, we dutifully returned wearing Chinese-made, counterfeit N95 masks (ironic, isn't it?), plastic face shields, double hand condoms, frilly shower caps, smelly rubber gowns and knockoff, disposable booties. It was the same type of knee-jerk, PPE reaction that we had in response to the AIDS epidemic during the early eighties. But what else could we present pikers do? Safety first but, in addition, unemployment insurance and government stimulus checks could only go so far and would run out anyway, sooner than later. I mean I could have stayed down on the fiscal mat if I had absolutely wanted to. I could have tightened my financial belt and tapped into my pension plan early but decided not to. Perhaps I'm being arrogantly foolish, but I believe that I might live a little longer and therefore keep on padding my monetary reserves by rote for that elusive future. It might work out, we'll see. In the meantime, I reluctantly chose to crawl back into the same nitty-gritty oral hellholes to chase those damn banknotes some more and to be eligible, once again, for employer-discounted health insurance. Although practicing part-time, I am ambivalently back in the saddle and dancing with the devil again. Once more I am restoring implants, making dentures, cutting enamel, and saving teeth. I'm continually plugging away while plugging endless cavitated teeth; still drillin' and fillin' for a livin'! And not surprisingly, that prophetic lyrical refrain still applies: same as it ever was. However, after that four-month layoff, this time I seem to have a better attitude, slightly thicker skin and more gratitude. I surmise I'll go at it for a little while longer, at least until Medicare and Social Security kick in unless competitive pickleball or a new and improved, foreign-born pestilence kills me first. As an aside, most dentists and necessary ancillary personnel finally got "The Vaccine" so Covid-19 should no longer pose a danger to us. Other Covid numbers, I'm not so sure about. But the way this country is going, perhaps we should ALL get a distemper shot as well. And now that we have an old, new president, let's look forward to a brighter future. However, lofty and idealistic rhetoric not rooted in realism often translates to failed promises and policies – same as it ever was? "Why, soitenly!" as Curly would say.

Disclaimer

I wish to apologize to all living and deceased patients, and dental staff whom I may have inadvertently denigrated, insulted or worse. Any resemblance of the people in my life to the characters, names and initials in this book was largely coincidental. And if you were a victim of circumstance or literary collateral damage, I am truly sorry. However, if you recognize yourself in any of the vignettes as the asshole that made my dental life miserable and a living hell, you had it coming. Turnabout is fair play; karma can be a real bitch. And I'm not kidding, or am I?

Last Words

You've made it this far and I thank you. I sincerely hope that some of you have had at least a few chuckles while reading this volume, and easily digested my oftentimes longwinded diatribes against the daily "grind" of dentistry and the patients who dehumanize it. But some of you thought it was funny, right? And hopefully some of you laughed at my "pain" as well! These forty unique episodes were culled from over thousands of anguishing yet mostly successful patient encounters, rendered treatments and dental experiences. Anyhow, here are a few salient takeaways from my often glib, snarky, sarcastic and harsh rhetoric demeaning the noble dental field and all who participate in it. Firstly, my long-suffering wife, Hottie Blondie, is fond of reminding me that dentistry was all MY idea; no one put a gun to my head making me apply to dental schools in the first place. Although maybe someone should have put a gun to my head to scare me out of doing it! Secondly, I hated pharmacy (my first vocation) as a job so that was a nonstarter. And lastly, let's say my love of insects garnered me an entomology Ph.D. after pharmacy college and I became a "bug" professor and researcher. Would I now be sick and tired of endless teaching responsibilities, stupid students and the ad nauseum curation of lifeless, pinned, six-legged carcasses? Perhaps it was just me, after all. What possible profession could I have chosen which would have made me reasonably wealthy, kept me relatively healthy and given me a modicum of self-respect? Not to mention ego boosting notoriety and the added bonus of being called a "doctor" to my face? And all without the blood and guts of medicine? That's right: dentistry! Plus, I was very good at it, at least that's what I was told in dental school. However, initially it seemed as though the bad far outweighed the good. I recently reflected on a long career full of unrealistic expectations, unwarranted malpractice suits, pro bono work (unintentional, of course), debilitating stress and "Aggravation Saturation." Did I really sacrifice sanity over lifestyle? Maybe so. Nevertheless, do I regret not being a pharmacist? Not on your Nellie! Am I thrilled at being a financially secure but abysmally aggravated dentist for over thirty-five years? Not on your Nellie! Even Doc Holliday left dentistry to pursue a life of gambling and gunfighting while in the throes of terminal tuberculosis. Was drilling humans with hot lead less stressful than drilling teeth? Evidently, yes, and I applaud his ballsy change of careers. Congrats to at least one burnout-suffering dentist from the late 1800s who decided to take decisive albeit deadly action! But then I cogitated some more and realized that I am still married, own two international beachfront vacation villas, successfully educated my two gifted and athletic kids, have a few real estate holdings, and managed to save a few pennies, and yet am still squawking! What the eff? I HAVE to be happy and satisfied, n'est-ce pas? However, can personal lives and careers become psychologically intertwined and inseparable? Of course. I knowingly made my professional dental bed years ago and have been voluntarily lying in a state of quiet desperation ever since. In other words, that simmering stew called dentistry has permeated my mental status outside the office as well. Perhaps other dentists feel differently and make the obvious dichotomy of work and play an easy affair. Unfortunately, I never quite fully mastered the concept of compartmentalization. In any event, dentistry has been largely responsible not only for my materialistic largess but for the freedom it gave me to create, recreate, procreate, and to live my "best" life. It wasn't ALL doom and gloom, although…. Sure, I could have worried a whole lot less, rolled with the punches a whole lot more and not taken things so personally. However, as previously and poignantly stated: perhaps it was just me? And maybe it was because I still fondly recall Henry V., a spry old man who was my patient in the 1990s. This *cool cat* would stroll in for his appointments with a spring in his step and enthusiastically greet my entire staff, while smiling from ear to ear. And he ALWAYS made a point of asking me about my personal life. Whenever I returned the favor he would say, "I feel great and am having a great day!" And he meant it. His cheerful outbursts and positive outlook on life instantly elevated the office's mood, even my own. But was that the way to be? Was he a sincere phony and armchair optimist? Do you have to fake it until you make it? Did he master tons of spiritual self-help books and now embodied those teachings? Or was he innately the real deal and somehow discovered the keys to happiness and fulfillment? I don't know but I remember really looking forward to his visits. Perhaps the secret to his contentment was making others feel good? But isn't that what dentistry is supposed to do for both the doctor and patient? If that's the case, then I guess I missed the boat somewhere along the line. In addition, some of my most trying patients did not get the memo, either. Oh, well. Anyway, the future of the past is now my present. Did things turn out as planned? It's hard to say. Should I have picked dentistry as a livelihood in the first place? Possibly. Did I indeed help thousands of patients with their oral needs? Obviously. But did I also sell my soul and peace of mind for a few doubloons and the trappings of a "successful" doctor? Probably. However, I will let YOU decide if I did the right thing.

Thanks for the read.

About the Author

Dr. I. Mayputz (not his real name) graduated with highest honors from high school, from pharmacy college and summa cum laude from dental school. After completing a master's degree in prosthodontics at a then prestigious institution, he embarked on his dental career in private practice. He once briefly toyed with the idea of earning a Ph.D. to become an actual entomologist, but ultimately decided on a dreadfully stressful albeit lucrative livelihood instead. In addition to being an elite master's athlete, published verbal artist, naturalist and part-time naturist, he is also known as a caustic wit and provocateur. He wrote this book to entertain family, friends, and any curious sod willing to *experience* life as a dentist.

For more alleged levity by Dr. I. Mayputz, please read:

Dental School: A Bizarre Comedy

Pharmacy College: Crazy Daze and Hazy Nites

Elementary School: Wits and Twits

Junior High: The Muddle Years

High School: Buffoonery Central

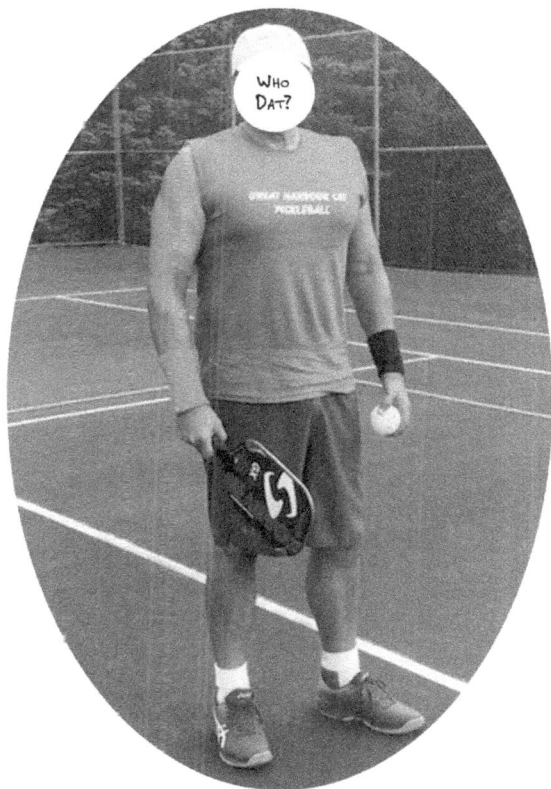